Management of Swallowing and Feeding Disorders in Schools

Management of Swallowing and Feeding Disorders in Schools

Emily M. Homer, MA, CCC-SLP

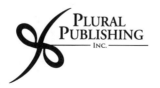

PLURAL
PUBLISHING
INC.

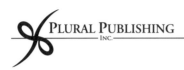
PLURAL PUBLISHING
INC.

5521 Ruffin Road
San Diego, CA 92123

e-mail: info@pluralpublishing.com
Website: http://www.pluralpublishing.com

FSC
www.fsc.org
MIX
Paper from
responsible sources
FSC® C011935

Typeset in 11/13 Garamond by Flanagan's Publishing Services, Inc.
Printed in the United States of America by McNaughton & Gunn, Inc.

For permission to use material from this text, contact us by
Telephone: (866) 758-7251
Fax: (888) 758-7255
e-mail: permissions@pluralpublishing.com

Every attempt has been made to contact the copyright holders for material originally printed in another source. If any have been inadvertently overlooked, the publishers will gladly make the necessary arrangements at the first opportunity.

NOTICE TO THE READER
Care has been taken to confirm the accuracy of the indications, procedures, drug dosages, and diagnosis and remediation protocols presented in this book and to ensure that they conform to the practices of the general medical and health services communities. However, the authors, editors, and publisher are not responsible for errors or omissions or for any consequences from application of the information in this book and make no warranty, expressed or implied, with respect to the currency, completeness, or accuracy of the contents of the publication. The diagnostic and remediation protocols and the medications described do not necessarily have specific approval by the Food and Drug administration for use in the disorders and/or diseases and dosages for which they are recommended. Application of this information in a particular situation remains the professional responsibility of the practitioner. Because standards of practice and usage change, it is the responsibility of the practitioner to keep abreast of revised recommendations, dosages, and procedures.

Library of Congress Cataloging-in-Publication Data

Homer, Emily M., author.
  Management of swallowing and feeding disorders in schools / Emily M. Homer.
    p. ; cm.
  Includes bibliographical references and index.
  ISBN 978-1-59756-515-8 (alk. paper)—ISBN 1-59756-515-6 (alk. paper)
  I. Title.
  [DNLM: 1. Child. 2. Deglutition Disorders—rehabilitation. 3. Adolescent. 4. Disabled Children—rehabilitation. 5. Feeding and Eating Disorders of Childhood. 6. School Health Services. WI 250]
  RJ206
  649'.151—dc23
                                                          2015022422

Contents

Foreword

I am privileged to be asked to write this foreword to *Management of Swallowing and Feeding Disorders in Schools*. This book is anticipated to become a major resource for speech-language pathologists (SLPs) and other professionals in a variety of school settings as they are increasingly being faced with children demonstrating a range of swallowing problems (dysphagia) as well as broader-based feeding problems. The American Speech-Language-Hearing Association has developed guidelines for SLPs that include knowledge and skills needed, roles and responsibilities, and also stresses the need for interdisciplinary teams. A major strength of this book is that it provides guidance in practical ways that cover a wide range of topics important to optimizing evaluation and intervention for these children, so they can function in their educational environments in the best ways possible.

Populations of children with swallowing and feeding disorders vary markedly. These children are in school settings. Many children have complex medical and surgical histories with varied severity of their conditions and changes expected over time. Thus, it is vital that professionals in the schools have extensive knowledge regarding underlying etiologies, nutrition, and health needs. Risks for aspiration must be considered in decision making, especially for children with underlying neurologic deficits. This book not only provides information in these areas, it also provides guidelines related to legal and ethical issues that must be taken into account for decision making by the school team and parents/caregivers working together for the best possible outcomes for all children to optimize school achievement and overall quality of life.

Chapter headings in this book cover the following topics: Addressing dysphagia in the school setting, legal issues, team approaches to identification and management, importance of safe swallowing, management processes preschool through 12th grade, children with behavioral and/or sensorimotor feeding disorders, addressing nutrition in the schools, working with parents/caregivers, and finally, training and competency issues in the schools.

All of this information is provided in a team approach that is vital to total care of every child with swallowing and feeding problems. Overall, this book is an important resource for all professionals working with children in the schools who deserve the best possible care in these areas that are critical as a foundation for all learning and experiences in life.

—Joan C. Arvedson, PhD, CCC-SLP, BC-NCD,
BRS-S, ASHA Fellow
Board Recognized Specialist in Swallowing and
Swallowing Disorders
Program Coordinator, Feeding and Swallowing
Services
Children's Hospital of Wisconsin-Milwaukee
Milwaukee, Wisconsin

Introduction

In 1995 my husband and I had our third daughter, Jojo, who was 11 and 16 years younger than our other two girls. I took a year sabbatical and during that year attended a Jeri Logemann presentation on dysphagia. When I returned to work the next year, I was curious about children with dysphagia in my school district. Three things happened that led my school district to form an interdisciplinary swallowing and feeding team.

1. A student's IEP came to my attention because it had a dysphasia goal (notice the misspelling) that was written by a classroom teacher. The goal stated that if the child starts choking to have her sit with her chin down and then give her coke. This child did not receive speech and language or occupational therapy services, so this was being written and implemented by a special education teacher. Obviously, at some point the student had been treated for dysphagia, but not unlike the childhood game of telephone where the message is changed by the time it gets back to the first child, the plan for addressing a choking situation had drastically changed over the years.

2. The second event that took place was when an elementary student in my district went on a class field trip (mother was chaperoning) and choked at McDonalds. After that incident, the mother informed the school for the first time that her son had a paralyzed vocal cord, and she wanted to know what the school was going to do if her child choked at school. We did not have a procedure in place to address this type of concern.

3. Finally, the third event, which occurred in 1996, was that the Medicaid cap for speech and language services went into effect, and some SLPs moved from working in the hospital setting to working in the schools. These SLPs with medical experience brought with them their skills, knowledge, and experience with dysphagia. They

recognized immediately that there were students in the
school setting who needed to be treated for swallowing
and feeding disorders who were at risk for aspiration.

The confluence of these events prompted us to form a committee to investigate identifying and treating dysphagia in the
schools and to come up with a procedure. We approached Jeri
Logemann at a presentation in New Orleans in 1998, and she
asked us to write an article on what we were doing for the
LSHSS dysphagia in the schools forum, published January 2000.
The SLPs in St. Tammany Parish Schools, Louisiana, along with
Occupational Therapists, Nurses, Physical Therapists, classroom
teachers, classroom paraprofessionals, cafeteria managers and
staff members, and school administrators and supervisors have
been working to help children eat safely at school since.

This book is based on the experiences that we have had for
the past 20 years identifying and treating children with swallowing and feeding disorders in the school setting. The procedure presented here has been shared with many school districts
throughout the country and has been successfully adapted,
tweaked, and personalized for each system based on their state
and local regulations, size of their district, and personnel available.

Each chapter addresses important information essential to
working with children with swallowing and feeding disorders in
the school setting and is designed to provide information which
will assist school teams. Chapter 1 is one of the most important
chapters because it tells the reader the process for establishing
a team in their district and for getting district approval. School
employees need commitment from the district that is provided
in a system-wide procedure. The following chapter covers the
importance of understanding legal, ethical, and regulatory issues
around this topic. This awareness allows school-based professionals to work with confidence knowing they are operating
within the law and ethics of each of their professions. The procedure is explained in Chapter 3 and provides the information
that district employees need to address swallowing and feeding
disorders using a multidisciplinary team. Subsequent chapters
provide information on identifying the disorder and utilizing
instrumental examinations, intervention with identified students,
and working with students with behavioral feeding disorders.

Finally, the book addresses the importance of nutrition in the school setting, working closely with parents/guardians and competency and training.

My mission and motivation for this work is for all school districts to recognize the importance of keeping all children safe at school when eating and drinking by establishing a system-wide procedure for addressing swallowing and feeding disorders. My goal is that school-based therapists and nurses have the information they need to be able to begin helping children with swallowing and feeding disorders in the schools as soon as possible!

Acknowledgments

The original group of SLPs, OTs, and nurses who in 1996 saw a need and worked together to come up with a procedure that would ensure that children could receive adequate nutrition and hydration while at school.

Carol Hillier and Sharon Hosch, Supervisors of Special Education in St. Tammany Parish Schools, who always put children first and supported this initiative from the beginning to the present.

Lennie Monteleone, past Superintendant of Schools in St. Tammany Parish, who believed in public education and encouraged us to share with other public districts the work we were doing.

Jeri Logemann who saw the importance of school-based SLPs addressing dysphagia. In 2000, she gave us our first platform for sharing the information through the LSHSS forum she was chairing on swallowing and feeding in the schools.

Joan Arvedson whose work has touched so many children and their families around the world. She is tireless in her mission to help us all understand the complex issues that are involved when working with children with swallowing and feeding disorders. Her guidance and advice helped me to understand that I could write a book on this topic and how it should be done.

Kim Priola who is my favorite person to collaborate with on issues related to swallowing and feeding in the schools and whose great ideas and hard work are reflected in this book.

Kristy Benefield, Patty Carbajal, Elizabeth Duncan, Chad Fabre, Crissy Faust, Sunny Johnson, Melissa Ogden, Kim Priola, and Roberta Torman for working to come up with a Behavioral Feeding Procedure to use in the school setting.

To school-based SLPs whose jobs are incredibly difficult and who have so much knowledge to give to students. Their knowledge, skills, and work are instrumental to the successful identification and treatment of swallowing and feeding disorders in the schools.

Contributors

Memorie M. Gosa, PhD, CCC-SLP, BCS-S
Assistant Professor
Department of Communicative Disorders
The University of Alabama
Clinical Affiliate
LeBonheur Children's Hospital
Tuscaloosa, Alabama
Chapter 4

Emily M. Homer, MA, CCC-SLP
Coordinator
Speech-Language-Hearing Therapy Program
St. Tammany Parish Public Schools
Covington, Louisiana
Chapters 1, 3, 5, 6, 7, 8, and 9

Lissa A. Power-deFur, PhD, CCC-SLP
Professor
Communication Sciences and Disorders
Director
Speech, Hearing and Learning Services
Longwood University
Farmville, Virginia
Chapter 2

This book is dedicated to my brother Joseph who helped to shape me and guided me to this field and to Greg, my love and support for two thirds of my life!!

1

Getting Started: Addressing Swallowing and Feeding in the School Setting

Emily M. Homer

Introduction

School districts around the country are recognizing the need to address swallowing and feeding disorders in students; however, many districts continue to question the educational relevance of working with swallowing and feeding and therefore choose not to address it. This book strives to be a resource to school-based personnel including speech-language pathologists, occupational therapists, school nurses, and others, as well as their districts as they go through the process of establishing a team procedure and managing and treating students with swallowing and feeding disorders. The primary goal and challenge with the management of swallowing and feeding (also referred to as dysphagia) in the school setting is ensuring that children eat, drink, and take medications safely while they are at school. Speech-language pathologists (SLPs) in the schools have many roles and responsibilities. Caseloads/workloads are high and their roles continue to

1

expand with new education initiatives such as Response to Intervention, co-teaching, and Value Added models. Dysphagia identification and treatment takes on educational relevance when it prevents a student from participating in their academic program to their fullest. This book helps school-based SLPs and other school-based professionals navigate working with students who have swallowing and feeding disorders in their school districts.

This chapter helps districts organize and design an interdisciplinary team procedure for addressing swallowing and feeding disorders. It begins by defining the disorder and connecting it to school systems by identifying the educational relevance of addressing swallowing and feeding according to the Individuals with Disabilities Education Act (IDEA). Speech-language pathologists, OTs, and nurses work with patients with swallowing and feeding disorders in a variety of medical settings. This chapter identifies, compares, and contrasts working with dysphagia in the school setting as compared to medical settings.

In addition, this chapter guides the reader through the process of getting administrative approval for a system-wide swallowing and feeding team procedure. There are several steps to accomplishing this task that are shared, including organizing a committee, going through the committee process, and preparing a proposal. Finally, this chapter guides the reader through selecting a team model based on the size and resources of the district and the management requirements of implementing the procedure.

What Are Swallowing and Feeding Disorders and What Are Their Implications in the School Setting?

The medical term used in hospitals, nursing homes, and skilled nursing facilities is dysphagia. According to the American Speech-Language-Hearing Association (ASHA), dysphagia is defined as "a swallowing disorder." The signs and symptoms of dysphagia may involve the mouth, pharynx, larynx, and/or esophagus" (ASHA, 2001). Taken from the ASHA Guidelines for speech-language pathologists providing swallowing and feeding services in the schools, ASHA documents have adopted "swallowing and feeding disorders" as the more inclusive phrase for dysphagia and delays and/or disorders in the development of eating and drinking skills, which are common in varied pediatric populations. Swallowing and feeding include the introduction, preparation, transfer, and transport of food and liquid from mouth through esophagus into stomach. In addition, management of saliva and oral intake of medications are included. Swallowing and feeding disorders vary considerably in their characteristics and severity. Children may demonstrate choking and aspiration, oral sensorimotor impairments, maladaptive behaviors during eating, refusal to eat, and acceptance of a restricted variety of food and liquid. Anatomic, neurologic, and/or physiologic impairments may include, but are not limited to, motor planning, postural control and oral-pharyngeal motor skills, sensory processing, respiration, and digestion. Students with severe disorders may experience deficiencies in nutrition and hydration, as well as reduced respiratory health (ASHA, n.d.).

Dysphagia refers to an interruption in the well-coordinated activity of the oral cavity, the pharynx, and the esophagus that includes the act of chewing and preparing food for the swallow, transporting the food through the pharynx down to the esophagus where the food enters the stomach. When a person has dysphagia they may have difficulty eating a normal diet and require some accommodations, strategies, and in some cases, therapeutic intervention to provide them with a means to acquire nutrition and hydration in a safe manner. Many of the cases that are seen in the school setting are oral phase dysphagia, which breaks down into the oral preparatory phase and the oral transit phase. Many children have weakened and compromised oral motor skills, which results in minimal and/or ineffective chewing skills. The lack of tongue lateralization, weak jaw movements, and immature chewing patterns, put these children at high risk for choking on food that is not ready for the oral transit phase, which then goes into the pharyngeal phase. In the pharyngeal phase there is a danger that the food and/or liquid will enter the airway and go into the lungs (aspiration) or blocks the airway. These issues necessitate addressing oral motor skills as well as altering food presentations and training school staff in the Heimlich maneuver and Cardiopulmonary Resuscitation (CPR). This is a serious risk that requires the services of a trained professional in the diagnosis and treatment of dysphagia. The school-based SLP often has this training and can facilitate the diagnosis of the disorder, the steps necessary to ensure a safe swallow and the recommended diet for a balanced nutrition program. It is extremely important that the SLP along with other school-based personnel use their training and skills to set up plans to safely feed students at school.

Identifying and Treating Dysphagia: Comparison of Services in Medical and Educational Settings

SLPs are trained extensively on the anatomy, physiology, causes, identification, and treatment of dysphagia. Most coursework and practicum focus on the adult population where the majority of dysphagia cases are treated. Many SLP's graduate school practicum and job experience with dysphagia occurs in hospitals, nursing homes, long-term care facilities, and home health with adults. Therapists with this training and experience have the skills needed to address dysphagia in the school setting; however, setting specific training and continuing education will be necessary.

In order for SLPs and OTs to recognize that the skills they already use in the medical setting can also be used in the schools, it may be beneficial to compare the similarities and differences of identifying and treating dysphagia in medical settings compared to the educational setting. Although there are some important, major differences there are also many similarities, which assist SLPs and OTs trained to work in the medical settings to use their skills to work with children in the schools. It is important that the SLPs and OTs who have this experience recognize that the skills can transfer to the school setting. Children, like adults, may develop swallowing and feeding issues that they did not have before as in cases such as closed head injuries, some syndromes and neurological disorders. In most cases in the school setting, children experience developmental or neurological disorders that result in a failure to develop normal swallowing and feeding skills. They often have the potential to improve their swallowing and feeding skills through therapeutic intervention or to delay the progression of degeneration. As a result, the school-based SLP faces fewer cases of medically unstable individuals whose dysphagia is a result of health issues such as stroke or declining skills and more cases where the disorder is present at or immediately after birth. Their clients are often learning the skills that will allow them to function safely and efficiently within the school setting. However, many of the challenges are the same as in other settings. In the schools, the therapist relies on paraprofessionals to feed the students in much the same way certified nursing assistants (CNAs) are used in hospitals, nursing homes, and other medical-based settings. Food for students and patients alike is prepared in cafeterias where balanced, nutritious meals are often adapted and modified to meet the specific guidelines of a swallowing and feeding plan. The SLP is usually responsible for managing a client's dysphagia while working with other team members in all settings including the schools. The SLP monitors and adjusts the dysphagia plan and trains family members and staff to assist with safe feeding in all settings. Regardless of the work setting, the identification and treatment of dysphagia is a team effort that requires all team members to remain current in their training and knowledge.

Collaboration with medical personnel is essential in the treatment of dysphagia. The collaboration with medical personnel is more challenging in the school setting. School districts typically must rely on the parents/guardians to communicate with physicians. Districts need to get signed releases, in most cases, to receive and share information with a student's physician.

School nurses assigned to students with swallowing and feeding disorders can help facilitate communication with the physicians. Although most of the other settings have medical staff support on site, the school setting is very limited in access to medical professionals, especially physicians.

The identification and treatment of dysphagia by definition includes working with oral, pharyngeal, and esophageal phases, however, in the school setting dysphagia therapists are also faced with behavioral feeding disorders that often interfere with students' ability to receive adequate nutrition and hydration during the school day and may put them at risk for associated heath issues. It is often difficult to determine the cause of the behavioral feeding disorder and medical issues will need to be ruled out prior to treatment. They are often the result of sensory, motor and/or behavioral issues, which prevent the child from eating a normal diet.

In medical settings, dysphagia is one of the primary disorders facing the SLP; however, in the school setting it is a very small percentage of what the SLP does on a daily basis. This is a low-incidence disorder in the schools and the result is that SLPs do not have as much experience with the issues and concerns surrounding dysphagia. As a result, SLPs in the schools need ongoing training and support in the complex issues that are presented in students with dysphagia.

These similarities and differences identify how dysphagia is addressed in the school setting as compared to other settings and shape how the team can be successful in securing a safe and nutritious eating environment for children with swallowing and feeding disorders (Table 1–1).

System-Wide Dysphagia Procedure: Setting Up a Swallowing and Feeding Team in Your District

One of the biggest concerns for the speech-language pathologist and other swallowing and feeding team members in a school setting is the fear of liability and due process. Although dysphagia is a medically based disorder, in most cases, the school is not a medical facility with medical staff ready to respond to emergencies. This combination of a medical condition and an educational setting requires a commitment on the part of the school district to provide guidelines to school personnel that clarify what is expected of school staff members and how the identification and treatment of a student with dysphagia should be approached. The solution is a system-wide procedure for addressing swallowing and feeding disorders that provides employees the support of the school system when addressing these issues.

Getting a district to adopt a procedure can be done in a relatively short time period by a group of knowledgeable and determined professionals. By following the steps in this section, the school team or committee can present to their district supervisors all of the information needed to address swallowing and feeding. Using this information, the district can design a swallowing and feeding team procedure that matches the needs and structure of their school system.

Table 1–1. Comparison of Addressing Dysphagia in Medical Settings and the Educational Setting

School Setting	Medical Setting	Both School and Medical Settings
Typically the result of neurological disorders, such as cerebral palsy, syndromes, such as Down, developmental delays, and behavioral feeding disorders.	Typically the result of stroke, dementia, Parkinson's, and other adult-onset disorders.	Some disorders are degenerative and require frequent monitoring and adjusting of swallowing and feeding plans.
Most students with dysphagia are medically stable.	Many clients are medically unstable and are frequently recuperating from an illness.	Person responsible for the daily feeding of the clients is typically a trained support staff such as a paraprofessional/classroom assistant in the schools and certified nursing assistant in medical settings.
Dysphagia identification and treatment is a small percentage of the SLP's job.	Dysphagia identification and treatment is a large percentage of the SLP's job.	Cafeteria staff members prepare texture and liquid modifications.
Dysphagia teams rely on parents to communicate with physicians and obtain health history.	SLPs are able to communicate directly with patient's physicians and work with family members to gather additional information.	Dysphagia is approached in both settings by interdisciplinary teams.
Minimal on-site medical support.	On-site medical support.	SLPs serve as the primary professional managing the patient/students swallowing and feeding needs.
		Rely on prescriptions from physicians to modify diets and monitor health.

School districts throughout the country have policy and procedures manuals that outline exactly what school personnel are to do in specific situations. There are policies and procedures for disciplining students, taking students on field trips, dress codes, and much more. Special education departments may have their own procedural manual that addresses the many issues that are associated with working with special needs students. It is in the interest of the district, school-based personnel, students, and parents that a school system adopts a procedure for identifying and treating students with swallowing and feeding disorders.

Benefits of a System-Wide Procedure

There are significant benefits to a school system adopting a procedure that will be the protocol used throughout the district. Students receive the services they need to be successful in school throughout the district in a uniform, consistent, and efficient manner, reducing confusion and uncertainty that comes when school personnel are uncertain about how to address an issue. Each of the benefits of a system-wide procedure will be discussed and can be used to support the request for a swallowing and feeding team procedure to district supervisors.

School Staff Knows What to Do

A system-wide procedure allows teachers and school staff to know exactly what to do and who to contact, when a student that has swallowing and feeding issues is placed in their classroom. The procedure provides the necessary steps that, when followed, ensures that all team members are accountable for the student and that documentation of their efforts is on file. A well-designed procedure provides the classroom staff with a plan of action when they are concerned that a child is having difficulty eating at school. It removes the "guesswork" and guides the teacher to the school personnel who can help determine the student's needs.

Embedded in the district procedure is the clarification of the roles and responsibilities of school-based personnel in relation to swallowing and feeding. The identification and treatment of swallowing and feeding is always a team effort. The school-based team typically consists of the SLP, teacher, parents/

guardians, occupational therapist (OT), physical therapist (PT), school nurse, paraprofessionals, and school administrators. Each member of the team has an important part to play in ensuring that students are safe at school. In order for them to be effective, it is necessary that they know and understand their own role and the role of others in the identification and treatment of swallowing and feeding in the school setting. Each professional's role in the swallowing and feeding team procedure is discussed in Chapter 3.

Sets Standards of How to Function

School systems adopt specific policies and procedures in order to set standards for functioning within the system. These policies and procedures provide the consistency and accountability that is important when completion of a variety of tasks is required by numerous personnel (Homer, 2008). A detailed procedure ensures that school personnel all follow the same steps to provide a safe eating environment at school. Classroom staff and other swallowing and feeding team members have a standard of accountability and documentation that can be monitored. This consistency not only benefits the children but also the professionals working with the student.

Students Have Access to Free and Appropriate Public Education (FAPE)

Providing students with a safe environment at mealtimes during the school day protects the student's right to a Free and Appropriate Public Education (FAPE) and the district's compliance in providing FAPE. In order for students to access their curriculum and to participate academically and socially throughout their school day they must have adequate nutrition and hydration as well as a means of taking medications when necessary. It is important that a district have a process in place for addressing the issues around swallowing and feeding. When a child is fed improperly they are often sick and miss school. They may lack the stamina to make it through the school day, to attend to their lessons, or socialize with their peers. In addition, students who are afraid of aspiration or choking at school may have trouble focusing on their lessons.

Educational Relevance

The American Speech-Language-Hearing Association's Clinical Topics/Pediatric Dysphagia (ASHA, n.d.) clarifies the question of the educational relevance of addressing swallowing and feeding disorders in the school setting. Addressing swallowing and feeding disorders is educationally relevant and part of the school system's responsibility for the following reasons:

- Children must be safe at school. School districts have the responsibility to provide a safe environment for students at school. Children must be able to eat at school in a safe manner, which reduces the chances of choking and aspiration.
- Students must have adequate nutrition and hydration at school in order for them to access their curriculum. This is necessary for a child to be able to focus at school and to have the stamina to make it through the school day.
- Students must be healthy in order to be able to attend school. Children suffering from undernourishment, dehydration, aspiration, or pneumonia will not be able to attend school and may have frequent absences.
- Students need to be able to eat within the time allotted at school with their peers whenever possible. In order to do this they must develop the skills necessary for eating efficiently.

Student Profile: Educational Relevance

Bethany is a 6th-grade student in regular education. She rides the bus to school, sits with her friends, and talks when she gets to school. She participates in the school routine and changes classes every 50 minutes until lunchtime. At lunch she eats what she likes on the tray while visiting with friends. Bethany is able to come to school, attend to her teacher, do her class work, and interact with the teacher and her friends. At recess she spends the time talking with friends. After lunch she is well nourished and ready to complete her school day. She has the stamina to access her curriculum throughout the school day.

Establish a Planning Committee

The first step in designing a system-wide swall
ing team procedure is to establish a committee t
of professionals within the school district who will be able to
contribute their unique perspectives on the issues, concerns, and
solutions associated with working with students who are high
risk for having or developing swallowing and feeding disorders
(Homer, Bickerton, Hill, Parham, & Taylor, 2000). The committee
should be made up of:

- Professionals who are knowledgeable about swallowing
  and feeding, and who recognize what the issues are and
  what will need to be done to establish a procedure.
- A variety of personnel who bring with them different
  viewpoints and skills including knowledge of the classroom setting.
- Participant who is knowledgeable about the district's
  rules and policies as well as how the district functions
  and how things are adopted within the system.
- Professionals who can function with the "give and take"
  of working on a committee.
- Members who have a commitment to work actively on
  the committee until the task is completed.

The committee will need to prepare information that will
inform school personnel, including school system administrators,
on swallowing and feeding disorders in children (Homer, 2008).

Choosing Committee Members

Typical committee key stakeholders in the identification and
treatment of swallowing and feeding disorders in the school
setting include:

- Speech-language pathologist
- Occupational therapist
- Physical therapist
- Nurse
- Special education teacher
- Social worker

- Dietician
- School administrator
- Parents

Once a committee has been selected, it will be necessary for someone to chair the committee. This should be someone who has the leadership skills to run a committee meeting. They should be able to schedule and organize committee meetings, keep the meetings task oriented and focused, and move the committee in the right direction. The chair of the committee should have a passion for swallowing and feeding disorders in children and knowledge of dysphagia.

The Committee Process

To get started, the following steps are recommended:

1. Outline the structure within your district for getting procedures approved. There will be a chain of command that will need to be followed. The committee should begin with the most immediate supervisor and move up to the administrator responsible for procedural decisions. An example of the path that may be followed is:
   a. Coordinators of related services such as speech and OT
   b. Special education supervisor
   c. Assistant superintendent
   d. Superintendent
2. Prepare the proposal for the team procedure including
   a. Defining the problem
      i. Definition of swallowing and feeding disorders
      ii. Educational relevance of addressing dysphagia
      iii. Risks associated with these disorders
      iv. Populations at risk (see Summary Sheet 1, Who and What of Swallowing and Feeding Disorders in the Schools, at the end of the chapter)
   b. Estimating the district's status
      i. Estimate of the number of students at risk
      ii. Estimate of the costs associated with a swallowing and feeding team such as: personnel, train-

ing, instrumental evaluations, and materials and
equipment.
c. Identifying the solution
   i. Establishing a system-wide procedure
   ii. Choosing a team model for addressing the issues
     of swallowing and feeding disorders
   iii. Securing the management requirements of the
      team process

Preparing a Proposal

When presenting a new procedure to school system administrators, the committee will want the information to be organized in
a concise, clear format. Using a worksheet such as the Proposal
Worksheet (Box 1–1) will assist the committee with this process.

Defining the Problem

Once the committee has been established, the members work on
compiling the information that will be presented throughout the
process to the upper administrative staff in the school district.
When going through the process, never assume that others know
or understand what dysphagia is and why it is important that it
be addressed in the schools. Unless the supervisor or administrator has had a family member diagnosed with dysphagia, it is
unlikely that they will be familiar with the term, the risk factors,
or the causes. The committee will need to be prepared to explain
the following: swallowing and feeding disorders in children, the
signs and symptoms, the risk factors associated with the disorder, the educational relevance, and who is at risk for swallowing
and feeding disorders. The Who and What of Swallowing and
Feeding Disorders in the Schools, at the end of this chapter,
provides a brief summary page of information that may be presented throughout the process to those who are not familiar with
dysphagia. Committee team members will be responsible for
educating district administrators as well as school staff members
throughout the process. Administrators who understand the disorder and its effect on students while at school will then be able
to make informed decisions regarding the system's responsibility
to students with swallowing and feeding disorders.

Box 1–1. Proposal for Swallowing and Feeding Team District Procedure

Proposal Worksheet: Interdisciplinary Swallowing and Feeding Team District Procedure

School System Chain of Command

Coordinators (related services such as speech and OT):

_____   _____

Supervisors (special education, school nurses, etc.):

_____   _____

Assistant superintendent(s):

_____   _____

Superintendent:

_____

System-Wide Swallowing and Feeding Team Rationale

- System is compliant with providing FAPE for all students
- Educational relevance of school attendance, attention, and social functioning are addressed
- Procedure for address swallowing and feeding is constant system-wide
- Classroom staff is aware of the procedure
- Personnel is assigned to schools to ensure adequate staff for addressing swallowing and feeding
- Process for documenting the procedure is in place
- Issues and concerns are addressed through the established procedure

Choose a Team Model

School Based   Combination   Core Team   Contract Services

Number of students at risk within the school system: _____

If a school-based model or combination model is chosen, it will be necessary to compare lists of SLPs, OTs, and school nurses with the students and their schools to determine who will address the student's swallowing and feeding. If a Core Team Model is chosen then the committee will need to consider who the team members will be and will need to adjust caseloads to allow time for working with students with dysphagia.

List Trained Personnel and School Assignments

Schools with at-risk students: _____

Trained SLPs/schools: _____

OTs/schools: _____

Nurses/schools: _____

Assign Core Teams and Case Managers

Assign students to core team members, SLP, OT, and nurse. In most cases these will be the professional assigned to the school for other services as well as swallowing and feeding. Assign one of the core team members to serve as case manager.

School: _____

Core team members: _____

Case manager: _____

Going through this process will determine the personnel needs of the school system, which can later be presented to district supervisors.

Additional Expenses

Identify training needs in district: _____

Professional development: _____

Procedural training: _____

CPR/Heimlich training: _____

Instrumental Evaluations

Minimal expense: _____

Typically less than 1% of dysphagia students will need these. Most students have Medicaid or private insurance that covers cost.

Materials and Equipment

- Assistive devices (chairs, special bowls, dyson mats, cups, spoons, etc.)
- Therapy tools (NUK brushes, Toothettes, Z-Vibes, Chewy Tubes, etc.)
- Bullet blenders for pureeing food
- Other: _____

Solution: System-Wide Swallowing and Feeding Team Procedure

Components of system-wide procedure:

- Referral
- Parent/guardian interview
- Interdisciplinary observation of swallowing and feeding
- IEP conference or 504 meeting
- Swallowing and feeding plan
- Individualized health plan
- Referral for MBSS
- Training classroom staff
- Working with cafeteria staff
- Monitoring swallowing and feeding

Documentation of Procedure

Forms for each step in the procedure:

- Referral form
- Parent/guardian interview form
- Interdisciplinary observation form
- Swallowing and feeding plan/classroom staff training form
- Individualized health plan
- Pre MBSS/VFSS referral form
- Prescription for school meal modification
- Transfer of students
- Documentation of communication
- Release for sharing and receiving medical information

Management Requirements of a Swallowing and Feeding Team

An administrator should be assigned to manage the swallowing and feeding team to do the following:

1. Assign case managers
2. Collect data on students followed
3. Arrange instrumental evaluations
4. Manage the movement of identified students within the district
5. Organize and provide ongoing professional development for team members
6. Work with parents and administrators when there are concerns and issues

This should be someone who is already employed by the school system in an administrative role such as coordinator of speech and language, coordinator of related services, lead SLP, and so forth.

Committee suggestions for swallowing and feeding team administrative manager:

_____

_____

Estimating the District's Status

Estimating the Number of Students at Risk. Once the committee has a plan for defining the problem and educating the district's administrators and school staff, they will need to estimate the number of students currently in their district who have the signs and symptoms of a swallowing and feeding disorder. Therapists, special education teachers, nurses, and other relevant workers should be given a referral form (see Appendix A) to complete on any student who they have observed the signs and symptoms of swallowing and feeding disorders. Special education teachers who work with students in the following populations should be given the referral form: severe/profound, mild/moderate, preschool early intervention, and autistic. These completed forms are returned to the committee members and the members with the training and experience in swallowing and feeding go to the schools and observe the students referred to determine if they are at risk. This accomplishes two things:

1. Identification of the number of students who are currently enrolled in the district who may need swallowing and feeding services.
2. Names of students who currently are at risk for complications related to swallowing and feeding disorders.

This information will be used to support the need for establishing a district supported swallowing and feeding team and to begin the task of ensuring that students in the district are safe during the process. School districts have the responsibility to ensure the safety of children at school. A district, including their employees, cannot do anything that they know will harm a child. Once a knowledgeable SLP, OT, or other professional has identified a swallowing and feeding need that has the potential of harming a child at school, then the district has a responsibility to address the issue. This somewhat complicates the process because, at the same time that the committee is working on getting district approval, they will be required to actually work with the students and their families/guardians to ensure their safety. It is suggested that the committee work quickly and efficiently to prepare the proposal and to begin the conversation with immediate supervisors so that they are aware of this ethical and legal requirement. It should also be noted that within this book is the general, big picture information that the committee will need to prepare the proposal. Using this information will expedite the process; however, the committee will need to adapt the information in this book to fit the particular requirements of their district and state.

Estimate of the Costs Associated With a Swallowing and Feeding Team. The district administrators will want to know the expenses associated with a swallowing and feeding team procedure. This section addresses the projected areas of expense but the amounts will depend on the size of the district and the personnel employed. The risks involved in a district not addressing swallowing and feeding could potentially be more expensive than the costs of implementing the procedure. School districts have the responsibility to ensure the safety of their students at school and safety when eating meals at school are included in that responsibility. A lawsuit could potentially cost the district a significant amount of money. In order to estimate the potential costs of addressing dysphagia, the committee will need to look at the following areas:

1. Personnel: The school-based interdisciplinary team may include the following professionals: SLP, special education teacher, OT, PT, nurse, paraprofessional, school administrator, social worker, and cafeteria manager. School districts in most cases already employ most of the professionals listed. When looking at a district's schools, every school should have a designated team of professionals who are trained in the procedure. In many cases these may be professionals already assigned to each school. The teacher, OT, PT, nurse, cafeteria manager, and others at each school may be designated as members of that school's swallowing and feeding team. The one exception is the SLP. In most cases, the SLP will be the primary case manager of the student being followed by the swallowing and feeding team. Each district will need a plan for ensuring that there is a trained SLP who can serve the students with swallowing and feeding disorders at each school. SLPs who have had

coursework and practicum and/or experience in the identification and treatment of dysphagia, regardless of the setting, are qualified to serve as swallowing and feeding team case managers. School districts that have many trained SLPs will be able to implement the swallowing and feeding team model without additional staff. Dysphagia is a low-incidence disorder in the schools (less than 1% of the district student population and 3% of the special education population) and in most cases can be added to the job description of the professionals involved without hiring additional staff. In many cases this may be accomplished by restructuring caseloads/ workloads or by hiring an SLP to serve as the district case manager. In some cases where there are no or very few trained SLPs, the district may need to add personnel to address swallowing and feeding. At this stage of the process, the committee will want to determine how many trained SLPs are employed in the district and select a model for addressing swallowing and feeding that utilizes the staff available. In many cases, by using one of the suggested models, districts are able to address swallowing and feeding without the expense of adding staff. The final personnel consideration is the assignment of a lead therapist or coordinator to address the district management of the interdisciplinary teams. Districts that already have Speech and Language Department Coordinators or Lead Therapist could add this task to their duties.

2. Training Costs: There are three types of training that will be necessary for the implementation of a district-wide swallowing and feeding procedure.

   a. Professional Development: The first type of training that will be needed is professional development in the area of pediatric swallowing and feeding. The main personnel who will be responsible for decision making with students with dysphagia, such as SLPs, OTs, and nurses, will need to continue to learn about the disorder, its implications with children, and current research. Training expenses will depend on the level of staff the district already employs. If a district has a large number of dysphagia trained SLPs and experienced OTs then much of the training can be in house. In any case some funds will need to be designated to send those responsible for identifying and treating swallowing and feeding disorders to professional development in their area to remain current and knowledgeable. In addition, each professional has a personal responsibility to stay current in their field of study, which results in them improving, expanding, or maintaining their skills. For example, nurses may choose to do research, reading, and training in the medical complications associated with swallowing disorders. OTs may direct their mandatory professional development requirements for licensure to research, reading and training in the areas of positioning, sensory integration and feeding skills. The school system may also provide professional development that is specific to addressing swallowing and feeding disorders in the pediatric population or in the school setting.

b. Procedural Training: Once a system-wide procedure is adopted, the district has a responsibility to ensure that all employees involved follow the procedure with fidelity. This will involve training classroom teachers, paraprofessionals, nurses, and others on the steps of the procedure and how to implement it, the roles of all of the team members, and the proper documentation of the procedure. School-based staff members such as teachers and paraprofessionals/ classroom assistants will need some general information on swallowing and feeding disorders, what they are, the signs and symptoms, and the complications (See Summary Sheet 1). This training should be done by the swallowing and feeding case manager, which is typically the SLP assigned to the case. Each person will need to be aware of their role on the team, what is required of them, what to look for, and how to react when they have a concern. It is beneficial for the teachers and paraprofessionals in the classroom to understand the basic anatomy and physiology of the swallowing mechanism and the complications that can occur when students with swallowing disorders are fed incorrectly. This type of training will require minimal expenses and can be done within the classroom setting. The district initially may decide to train teachers and paraprofessionals as a group, which may require substitutes or after-school stipends.

   c. Cardiopulmonary Resuscitation and Heimlich Maneuver: The final training involves cardiopulmonary resuscitation (CPR) and the Heimlich maneuver, which, in many cases, is already a requirement for continued employment with special education teachers and paraprofessionals. Classroom staff directly responsible for feeding children with dysphagia should annually receive CPR training. The district may leave the responsibility for this training to each individual or may provide the training. Some districts have nurses on staff who are trained as CPR trainers and are able to train district staff in house with the expenses limited to substitutes when done during the school day or stipends if after school.

3. Instrumental Evaluations: When estimating the cost of an interdisciplinary dysphagia team, it is necessary to allow some funds for instrumental evaluations such as modified barium swallow studies (MBSS)/videofluoroscopic swallow studies (VFSS) or Fiberoptic Endoscopic Examination of Swallowing (FEES) tests. The majority of children in the school setting with swallowing and feeding disorders have oral phase dysphagia and will not need to be referred for instrumental swallow studies; however, in a small number of students the district may request a referral from a physician for a swallow study. Students frequently have Medicaid or private insurance, which covers most of the expenses. According to IDEA school districts are responsible for medical evaluations and diagnosis, however, the school district is typically the payer of last resort, which frequently results in the district paying the co-pay or nothing (IDEA, 2004).

4. Materials and Equipment: Finally, the committee should estimate a small amount of money to cover materials

and equipment needed for some students with swallowing and feeding concerns. This expense typically comes out of the IDEA budget and includes items such as: adaptive/assistive feeding equipment including suction bowls, maroon spoons, and Infafeeders, therapeutic tools such as NUK brushes, Z-vibes, Toothettes, and Chewy Tubes, as well as food processors for texture alteration and protective gloves.

Identifying the Solution

Once the committee has gone through the process of identifying the problems and issues, estimating the costs, and determining the needs within the school system, they need to indicate to district administrators the solutions. The committee needs to outline the action plan for establishing a functional team within the system, including a suggested procedure, structure of team(s), and administration of the program.

System-Approved Procedure

A system-approved or district-approved procedure provides school staff members with the information they need to identify students who are at risk for swallowing and feeding problems, determine their swallowing and feeding needs and recognize when their needs change. This allows a school district to be proactive in ensuring that students are safe at school when they eat or drink. The committee should provide the district administrator a well-organized proposal for accomplishing the task. Box 1–1 assists the committee in preparing the proposal.

Components of a System-wide Procedure. A swallowing and feeding procedure in a school setting will need to be comprehensive and cover all pertinent areas. Listed below are the components of the actual procedure. Each step is explained in Chapter 3.

- Referral
- Parent contact and interview
- Interdisciplinary observation of the student eating
- Pre-IEP conference
- Swallowing and feeding plan

- Individualized health plan
- Diet orders from physician
- Cafeteria procedure
- IEP conference
- Medical referral for instrumental swallow study
- Revision of swallowing and feeding plan and/or individualized health plan
- Therapeutic intervention if indicated
- Monitoring of swallowing and feeding skills

In addition to the components of the procedure for identifying and addressing swallowing and feeding disorders in the schools, it is also necessary to have a process in place for the following:

- Assigning case managers to identified students
- Keeping track of students who are followed by the team
- Transferring students from school to school
- Discharging students from the swallowing and feeding team

Having a procedure in place that addresses the above areas will ensure that the school system is ready to address the complex issues and concerns that students with swallowing and feeding concerns often come upon.

Choosing a Team Model

There are several ways that a system can address swallowing and feeding in the schools. They all should involve an interdisciplinary team approach. The model of how a system chooses to address swallowing and feeding students will depend on the resources available. Each system needs to determine how they can best utilize the personnel who they already have on staff. Every school system is different and therefore every team approach will be a little different as well. Summary Sheet 2, Models for Addressing Swallowing and Feeding Working as a Team, outlines the different team models.

School-Based Team. The school-based team model is used when a system has trained SLPs, OTs, and nurses assigned to every school where the swallowing and feeding students attend. The swallowing and feeding needs of the students are addressed completely by core interdisciplinary team members who are also based at the school site and are addressing the other needs of the students at that school. This team model requires that a system have an adequate number of trained personnel to serve all of the students at their home school and it is the ideal model. The benefit to the school-based model is that the team members are part of the school staff, are familiar with the school, the students, and the teachers. This facilitates regular monitoring of the students and allows for more-involved swallowing and feeding therapy, if needed. The team members are able to interact more frequently with the other school staff as well as with parents/guardians. It also allows for collaboration of team members and for co-treating in some cases. Finally, it is beneficial when possible to have the professional who is most knowledgeable about a student's swallowing and feeding on the campus should an emergency occur. Few school districts have the trained personnel to implement this model and ongoing training with a large number of therapists and nurses can be challenging.

System Core Team. In some cases a school system will have a minimum number of professionals on staff who are trained and experienced in the identification and treatment of children with swallowing and feeding problems. These districts are often small and/or located a distance from university programs. A district with limited personnel may consider the system core team model. This model is composed of an SLP, OT, and school nurse all of whom have training with swallowing and feeding. This core team specializes in working with students with swallowing and feeding issues. They travel to the various school sites to serve the students with swallowing and feeding concerns. The team works collaboratively with the school-based personnel including the teacher, administrator, school-based SLP, OT, and nurse. The core team is responsible for following the procedure once a student is referred to the team. They establish the safe feeding plan and train the school staff to implement the plan and to report concerns and changes in the student's swallowing and feeding. The core team will want to set a schedule to visit each school according to the needs of the students. The school-based personnel such as the SLP and OT can be trained on the plan to assist with monitoring. The benefits to the system core team model is that the core team members work with more students with dysphagia and as a result develop more experience and knowledge. Fewer team members make ongoing training and staff development easier. This model has been successfully used in districts and is often a good option.

Combination Team Model. This team model works well for districts that have some schools with dysphagia-trained SLPs and some schools without dysphagia-trained SLPs. With the combination team model most teams are school-based, which allows the person most knowledgeable to be on campus and have all of the benefits of the school-based team model. In the schools where it is not possible to assign a dysphagia trained SLP, then a system core team serves the students at those schools with swallowing and feeding disorders. The core team works closely with the school personnel. As the district hires new SLPs, this model moves closer to the school-based model. The system may consider training and experience with swallowing and feeding disorders when hiring SLPs and OTs for schools where there is this need. The combination team model allows therapists with training and experience in swallowing and feeding disorders to use their skills and has all of the benefits of the school-based for some of the schools.

Contract Services. Some school districts do not have any trained or experienced SLPs or OTs. In this case, a school system may choose to contract with a private consultant or therapy group. The extent of the services provided by the consultant will depend on the number of cases, the severity of the cases and ability of the district to work toward training their school staff. If contract services are utilized it is important that they be ongoing. The consultant will need to identify the issues, set up safe swallow plans, train school staff, and then monitor the students on a regular basis. A system may choose to begin with contract services and work toward the core team model by hiring trained personnel.

School Building Level Team (Pilot Model). There are times when a school system will refuse to adopt a procedure. In these cases,

SLP, OTs and nurses are often in the situation where they have a child who needs these services but their district does not currently support addressing swallowing and feeding or is not aware that there is the need. In these cases, it is sometimes possible for a school to establish a procedure to be used with the students who attend that school. In this case, the SLP may have knowledge and experience in dysphagia and works with the school administration, OT, nurse, and so on to develop procedures to work with the swallowing and feeding cases at that school. The school district at large may not have a formal process or procedure in place but the school building base model (similar to a pilot program) may begin at the school level, which may lead to development of district policies. SLPs, OTs, and other professionals should only implement the school building team procedure when the school administration is part of the team and supports the procedure.

Referral Source. In cases where the therapeutic staff receives no support on a system level or when a school system is working on establishing a procedure the SLP, OT, and/or school nurse may work with parents to obtain an outside referral. In this case, however, the SLP, OT, and/or nurse will still have a responsibility to provide safe-feeding procedures to the classroom staff to ensure that the student is safe at school. The school administrator, special education administrator and district administrator should be notified of the situation.

Management Requirements of the Team Process

Whether in a large school district or a small one it is necessary for someone to manage the swallowing and feeding team(s) at a district level. An administrator, lead therapist, or core team leader, should be assigned to manage the swallowing and feeding team(s). The tasks that are required are the same but how they are managed will differ from system to system. The tasks that require a swallowing and feeding team administrator are summarized for quick reference in Table 1–2.

Assign Case Managers. It is important to have one member of the swallowing and feeding team be assigned case manager for

Table 1–2. Seven Duties of the Administrative Manager of the Swallowing and Feeding Team

1. Assign case manager to each student.

2. Track students followed by the swallowing and feeding team.

3. Arrange for instrumental evaluations when indicated.

4. Purchase materials and equipment for implementing swallow plan and therapeutic intervention.

5. Organize and provide ongoing professional development for team members.

6. Provide support and organize networking for therapists and nurses.

7. Work with parents/guardians and administrators when there are concerns and issues.

each child. In a small district where there is a core team, one of the core team members should be designated as the swallowing and feeding team coordinator. This person would then assign cases for each of the core team members to manage. In larger districts, this role becomes even more important because there are more children, schools, and swallowing and feeding team members to manage. The system administrator who is often the Coordinator of Speech and Language Programs or Lead Therapist, would receive the referrals from all cases at all of the schools. Once the referral is received, the system administrator designates the case manager for that student. In districts where the school-wide or combination team models are being used, the system administrator would designate at the beginning of each school year the case managers for each school. This should be done even for schools where there currently are no students being followed. In the course of the year, if a student is identified or transfers in, then there is a case manager in place who can begin working with the student immediately. Because of the nature of the disorder it is essential that each step move very quickly and efficiently. A student, once identified as needing swallowing and feeding services, must receive them immediately. See Table 1–3 for a sample Case Manager Assignment worksheet.

Table 1–3. Form to Assign Swallowing and Feeding Team Case Managers

Assignment of Swallowing and Feeding Team Case Managers			
School District Name:			
School Year:			
School	**Case Manager**	**School**	**Case Manager**
For example: Abita Elementary	Mary Smith	Lake Elementary	Kathy Smith Joan Miller

Note. A case manager should be assigned to every school in the district in the event that a student is identified with swallowing and feeding issues. In some larger schools it is possible to have two or more SLPs and/or OTs who may serve as case manager.

Tracking Students Followed by the Swallowing and Feeding Team. The system administrator should keep a data spreadsheet to track all of the students in the district who are being followed by the swallowing and feeding team(s). A copy of the Swallowing and Feeding Team Referral Form (see Appendix A) should be keep in a central location, along with updated swallowing and feeding plans (see Appendix B), transfers in and out of schools or the district (see Appendix C) and discharges from the school-based swallowing and feeding services. Fidelity in implementing the swallowing and feeding procedure is essential and the swallowing and feeding administrator is in the position to monitor implementation of the plans and documentation of the procedure.

Arrange Instrumental Evaluations. Addressing swallowing and feeding in the schools always includes working as an interdisciplinary team. The medical team members, although not part of the school system, are essential members of the team. Regular contact with the student's physician is recommended to ensure that the physician is kept informed of the student's swallowing and feeding status at school. Some student's swallowing status indicates the need for an instrumental evaluation such as a MBSS/VFSS or FEES. In these cases the district will need an administrator or designated clinician or nurse to facilitate the request for a physician's referral for these evaluations. In cases where the district assumes financial responsibility for the MBSS or FEES evaluation, it may be more efficient for the school system to set up the study directly with the hospital, including instructions that the school system will cover the cost of the study that is not covered by private insurance or Medicaid (Homer, 2008). This facilitates payment if it becomes necessary. In cases where the school system is requesting the study, the financial responsibility lies with the district. Having an administrator or designated person available for setting up these evaluations, receiving the reports, and insuring payment allows the procedure to flow more easily. It also allows for the student's swallowing and feeding case manager to attend the study with the child and parents/guardian.

Purchase Materials and Equipment. Implementation of a swallowing and feeding plan often requires specific adaptive equipment to assist the child in being successful during mealtimes. In addition, students receiving oral motor therapy and feeding therapy may need materials to use during therapy. The swallowing and feeding administrator is responsible for ordering both adaptive equipment and therapeutic materials.

Organize and Provide Ongoing Professional Development for Team Members. Team members need ongoing professional development and training in the procedure, issues, and research around swallowing and feeding disorders in children. The district swallowing and feeding administrator is responsible for organizing ongoing training. The district may sponsor their own professional development or may fund sending therapists and nurses to outside training.

Provide Support and Networking for Therapists and Nurses. Swallowing and feeding disorders in the schools can be very complex. A district should have in place a system that provides support for therapists as they navigate a student's swallowing and feeding, as well as, a process for networking with therapists who have the most experience and training. The administrator serves as a resource to connect therapists and to provide guidance with difficult cases. For this reason, it is essential that the swallowing and feeding administrator have sufficient training and experience to serve is this capacity.

Work With Parents/Caregivers and Administrators When There Are Concerns and Issues. Few things are as emotional for a parent as providing nutrition and hydration to their child. Parents are essential members of the interdisciplinary team and are active in determining safe feeding at school. There are times when a parent/guardian's opinion is different from the school's team. The system administrator will serve as a mediator and support in cases where there are disagreements.

Tips for Going Through the Process

The following tips will help the committee members proceed through the process of establishing a system-wide procedure to address swallowing and feeding in their district:

- Do not assume that anyone within system administration knows what dysphagia is; its risks and implications. Be prepared to educate throughout the process.
- Establish a vision, maintain your vision but be willing to compromise throughout the process.
- Use the question, "Is it best for children?" throughout the process as a guide to decision-making.
- Follow your system's chain of command when presenting the concept of establishing a dysphagia team.
- Have an idea what the model will cost the system, but be ready to point out that it may prevent future due-process cases.
- Keep everyone involved, especially pertinent administrators, informed throughout the process.
- Always be prepared with information supporting the requirements for districts to address swallowing and feeding including the educational relevance and ethical responsibilities of school-based personnel.

Summary Sheet 1: Who and What of Swallowing and Feeding Disorders in the Schools

What Is a Swallowing and Feeding Disorder?

Swallowing and feeding disorders (also known as *dysphagia*) include difficulty with any step of the feeding process—from accepting foods and liquids into the mouth to the entry of food into the stomach and intestines. A *swallowing or feeding disorder* includes developmentally atypical eating and drinking behaviors, such as not accepting age-appropriate liquids or foods, being unable to use age-appropriate feeding devices and utensils, or being unable to self-feed. A child with dysphagia may refuse food, accept only a restricted variety or quantity of foods and liquids, or display mealtime behaviors that are inappropriate for his or her age (ASHA, n.d.).

Who Is at Risk for Swallowing and Feeding Disorders?

Swallowing and feeding disorders occur in all age groups, from newborns to the elderly and can occur as a result of a variety of congenital abnormalities, structural damage, and neurological disease or disorder. Primarily those at high risk for a swallowing disorder in the school setting are those who may be identified as:

- Developmental disorders
- Cognitive deficits
- Cerebral palsy (CP)
- Traumatic brain injury (TBI)
- Neurological impairment
- Various syndromes
- Autism
- Cleft palate

continues

What Are Some of the Signs and Symptoms of a Swallowing and Feeding Disorder?

- Repeated respiratory infections/history of recurring pneumonia
- Poor oral motor functioning
- Maintains open mouth posture
- Drooling
- Nasal regurgitation
- Food remains in mouth after meals (pocketing)
- Coughing/choking during or after meals
- Weight loss/failure to thrive
- Refusal to eat
- Wet or "gurgle" voice/sound after meal
- Difficulty chewing

What Are the Complications of a Swallowing and Feeding Disorder?

- Aspiration (entry of food or liquid into the airway (trachea) below the true vocal folds that leads to the lungs.)
- Pneumonia
- Dehydration
- Undernutrition
- Choking

Educational Relevance for Addressing Swallowing and Feeding Disorders in the School Setting

According to IDEA, all students are entitled to a free and appropriate public education (FAPE). Health services are included in IDEA as a related service that helps to ensure FAPE. In order for a child to have FAPE, he or she must be healthy, well-nourished, and hydrated so that they can:

- Attend school
- Benefit fully from academic instruction
- Socialize with peers
- Efficiently complete mealtimes

Summary Sheet 2: Models for Addressing Swallowing and Feeding Working as a Team

Swallowing and Feeding Team Models Will Look Different Depending on the Make-Up of Your District

- School-based teams—team members who are assigned to the school make up that team's dysphagia team: SLP, OT, PT, nurse, etc.
- System core team—a separate team composed of an SLP, an OT, and school nurse who specializes in swallowing and feeding, travels to various school sites to serve students with dysphagia.
- Combination teams—district has some schools with dysphagia-trained teams on campus and some schools that rely on a system core team.
- Contract services—district contracts services with a private consultant when the district has no dysphagia-trained SLPs on staff.
- School building level team—an SLP in a specific school may have knowledge and experience in pediatric dysphagia and works with the building administration to develop procedures to work with dysphagia cases. The school district at large may not have a formal process/ procedure in place but the school building base model may begin at the school level and lead to the development of district policies by piloting the procedure.
- Referral source—an SLP in a school system receives no support on a building or district level but continues to work with parents to obtain an outside referral and provides the safest feeding procedures to the staff and documents this process

continues

School-Based Team Approach to Swallowing and Feeding

- The interdisciplinary approach involves each member of a group of professionals, each who brings a specific area of expertise.
- A true interdisciplinary approach involves each member of the group sharing the philosophy for diagnosis and treatment in addition to being willing and able to work with other team members within the group (Arvedson & Brodsky, 2002).
- Be aware of each person's role.
- Share information.
- Realize personal professional limitations in relation to dysphagia.
- Be open to suggestions and to problem solving.
- Have open communication among the team members.

Medical-Based Team

- Medical team members often include the following physicians: pediatrician, pulmonologist, gastroenterologist, ENT, and others.
- Access to a dietician.
- The hospital SLP—important to collaborate with the hospital SLP prior to the MBSS/VFSS.
- Radiologist—will work with you during the MBSS/VFSS.

When to Contact the Physician?

- When there is a serious concern about the student's health status
- To request a script for a Modified Barium Swallow Study/Videofluoroscopic Swallow Study
- To request a change in diet orders
- When there are concerns about a child's nutritional intake
- To get a more thorough medical history

References

American Speech-Language-Hearing Association. (n.d.). *Clinical topics/ pediatric dysphagia*. Retrieved June 15, 2015, from http://www.asha .org/Practice-Portal/Clinical-Topics/Pediatric-Dysphagia

American Speech-Language-Hearing Association. (2001). *Roles of speech-language pathologists in swallowing and feeding disorders: Technical report*. Retrieved from http://www.asha.org/policy

Arvedson, J., & Brodsky, L. (2002). *Pediatric swallowing and feeding: assessment and management* (Rev. ed.). San Diego, CA: Singular.

Homer, E. (2008) Establishing a public school dysphagia program: A model for administration and service provision. *Language, Speech, and Hearing Services in Schools, 39*, 177–191.

Homer, E., Bickerton, C., Hill, S., Parham, L., & Taylor, D. (2000). Development of an interdisciplinary dysphagia team in the public schools. *Language, Speech, and Hearing Services in Schools, 31*, 62–75.

Individuals with Disabilities Education Improvement Act of 2004, 20 U.S.C. § 1400 et seq. (2004).

2

Legal, Regulatory, and Ethical Considerations

Lissa A. Power-deFur

Introduction

As a school-based speech-language pathologist, you spend time in a variety of special education classrooms collaborating with teachers. Over the course of a few weeks, while collaborating with the classroom teacher in her early childhood special education classroom, you become concerned about a newly enrolled child who exhibits frequent coughing, choking, and gagging during mealtime and snack. You express your concerns to the teacher assistant who feeds the child. She states that this "always happens, even if I give him his favorite foods!" The assistant expresses frustration at how challenging it is to deal with the child's behavior during mealtime and that he refuses to eat anything except cheese puffs and chicken nuggets.

In the elementary special education classroom, you observe a newly enrolled child who has a significant intellectual disability and cerebral palsy. You note that the child is typically seated in a wheelchair and is often slumped to one side when the paraprofessional feeds her. When speaking with the aide, you learn that the child is frequently absent from school due to respiratory issues and occasional pneumonia. You know that symptoms of choking, coughing, and gagging, limited repertoire of food consistencies and textures, and respiratory issues may signal the presence of swallowing difficulties. As such, you become concerned that there are children with untreated dysphagia problems in your school.

These scenarios are examples of situations that school-based professionals may observe. They highlight the importance of school district personnel being knowledgeable in the area of swallowing and feeding including legal and ethical considerations.

The scope of practice in speech-language pathology and the American Speech-Language-Hearing Association position on roles and responsibilities of school-based speech-language pathologists provides a clear and distinct role for the provision of swallowing and feeding services for all populations (American Speech-Language-Hearing Association, 2007, 2010b). According to the American Speech-Language-Hearing Association (ASHA) Schools Survey (2012), 11% of school-based speech-language pathologists reported evaluating and treating children with dysphagia, with an average of 2.6 children on their caseload at any given time during the academic year. Speech-language pathologists working in day or residential schools and preschools report the highest level of children on their caseload receiving dysphagia services (41.2% and 20.5%, respectively), followed by speech-language pathologists working in elementary (8.4%) and secondary schools (5.4%). These figures are in contrast to data reported by Castillo, Carr, and Nettles (2010), who found that 17% of children under age 18 and who have a developmental disability require a food substitution or modification in the school nutrition program. Moreover, Cerezo, Lobato, Pinkos, and LeLeiko (2011) stated that 25% to 35% of normally developing children and up to 80% of children with neurodevelopmental disabilities may have feeding and swallowing problems. Unfortunately, many of these children may be either unserved or underserved in public education due to confusion amongst speech-language pathologists and others regarding how swallowing and feeding services align with the academic expectations of public education. This chapter: (a) provides background information surrounding special education statutes and regulations, special education case law related to children with health care needs, including dysphagia, and Medicaid funding for special education services; (b) addresses ethical issues in the provision of services to children with dysphagia; and (c) offers recommendations for practice to assist school-based speech-language pathologists and school districts as they address the needs of children with dysphagia.

Special Education Requirements

Many speech-language pathologists find that their school districts don't view swallowing and feeding as a special education service. A review of the focus of federal special education statues and regulations assists in understanding this point of view. In 1975, Public Law 94-142, the Education for All Handicapped Children Act (EAHCA) was enacted "to assure that all children with disabilities have available to them . . . a free appropriate public education that emphasizes special education and related services designed to meet their unique needs" (20 U.S.C. 1401(a)(9)). A free appropriate public education (FAPE) is based on the provision of special education and related services to eligible students. It is important to remember that P.L. 94-142 was first enacted based upon the principle of civil rights for persons with disabilities—to ensure equal access to public education for children with disabilities and prohibit disability discrimination.

The law focuses on instruction, stating that children with disabilities must receive "specially designed instruction" in order to meet their unique needs (34 CFR §300.39(a)(1)). The parameters of special education law have evolved significantly in the past four decades, through reauthorization of the Act (currently titled the Individuals with Disabilities Education Improvement Act of 2004 [IDEA]) (Individuals with Disabilities Education Improvement Act , 2006) federal regulations, state laws and regulations, and case law. These iterations of the statute and the regulations implementing it have defined parameters regarding the services that are provided. In addition, recent reauthorizations and the interrelationship of IDEA, with the expectations for student achievement found in No Child Left Behind, have further raised the academic expectations for students with disabilities.

IDEA is a funding law that mandates state compliance in order to receive federal special education funds. IDEA delegates the responsibility to develop implementation regulations and policies and the authority to assure compliance with the federal law and regulations to the states. State legislatures also have the authority to pass statutes and direct development of regulations that are related to public education. Although these state-level statutes and regulations largely affect general education, they also have an effect on the education of children with disabilities. State laws and regulations may not supersede federal requirements, but can have a significant effect on requirements not addressed federally (e.g., special education timelines, graduation requirements). With 50 states, there are 50 different variations to selected aspects of the special education requirements and interpretations.

Public education in the United States is ultimately the responsibility of local government, with federal involvement only occurring within the last 50 years. Therefore, the final authority for establishment of education policies and procedures, including those affecting students in special education, rests with local school districts and their governing bodies (e.g., local school boards). Each school district establishes its own policies and procedures for implementation of the federal and state requirements in order to ensure compliance, and to potentially prevent due process hearing and lawsuits. The local autonomy given to school districts further contributes to the variability of special education policies and procedures across the country. As a result, there may be vast differences in implementation from state-to-state and district-to district.

The Special Education Process

IDEA establishes a process for identifying and providing services to children with disabilities. Special education services are provided to children who, through an assessment process, are identified by an eligibility team as meeting the criteria to be identified as a "child with a disability." The three criteria are: (a) the child has a disability identified by IDEA (e.g., speech-language impairment, orthopedic impairment, other health impairment); (b) the disability has an adverse educational impact on the child's ability to progress in the general curriculum; and (c) the child will benefit from receiving special education and related services. Education professionals complete a variety of assessments to understand the nature of the child's disability. The eligibility team—a team of educators and the parent(s)—reviews the assessment reports and information about the child's performance in the general curriculum. In addition to evaluation results, the team also considers the observations conducted in the classroom and teacher reports. These data serve to inform the committee's decision as to whether the child meets any of the federal definitions of disability and if the presence of disability may adversely affect the child's education.

IDEA establishes categories of disabilities that describe children who are eligible to receive special education and related services. IDEA defines a speech-language impairment as follows: "a communication disorder, such as stuttering, impaired articulation, a language impairment, or a voice impairment that adversely affects a child's educational performance" (IDEA, 34 CFR §300.8 (c)(11)) (IDEA, 2006). This definition was crafted in 1975 when dysphagia was not regarded as a part of the speech-language pathologist's scope of practice. The Act has been reauthorized many times over the last three decades; yet, dysphagia has not been included as part of the definition. However, in its review of comments on the regulations supporting IDEA in 2007, the U.S. Department of Education considered adding dysphagia. It declined to do so, citing "we believe that the definition is sufficiently broad to include services for other health impairments, such as dysphagia" (Assistance to States, 2006). However, as children with dysphagia have multiple disabilities, specialized health needs, and/or are medically fragile, it is unlikely that a child with dysphagia would be found eligible for special education solely under the category of speech-language impairment.

The focus of IDEA is on education. As such, its purpose is to assure equal access for children with disabilities to the educational system. IDEA's eligibility criteria make clear that all children who have a disability may not be eligible to receive special education. Although a child may have a disability, the assessment results may not indicate an adverse educational impact or the need to receive special education and related services. When considering the adverse educational impact, however, the eligibility team must consider other factors in addition to classroom performance. For example, if the child's disability prevents the child from attending or participating in school, then these additional factors may also have an adverse impact on education. This consideration is particularly important for students with other health impairments, including those with swallowing and feeding disabilities.

The third eligibility criterion is whether the child needs to receive special education and related services. Special education is defined as specially designed instruction that meets the unique needs of a child with a disability, with a focus on enabling the child to access the general curriculum. The statute also states that students who are identified as eligible for special education may also receive related services. Related services include "transportation and such developmental, corrective, and other supportive services . . . as may be required to assist a child with a disability to benefit from special education" (34 CFR § 300.34(a)). Specifically, related services include speech-language pathology, physical and occupational therapy, and school health services. It is important to note that this list is illustrative rather than exhaustive. The Act specifies that the related service must be necessary for a child with a disability to benefit from special education. This requirement clarifies that although a child may benefit from a related service, unless the related services is needed for the child to benefit from special education, that related service is not the purview of IDEA.

The delineation between medical services and school health services can often be confusing for school-based teams. IDEA identifies medical services as those procedures that are for "diagnostic and evaluation purposes only" (34 CFR § 300.34(a). The definition of medical services further clarifies that the services are those provided by "a licensed physician to determine a child's medically related disability that results in the child's need for special education and related services" (34 CFR § 300.34(c)(5)). IDEA 2004 added school nurse services to the definition of school health services, indicating that: "school health services and school nurse services means health services that are designed to enable a child with a disability to receive FAPE as described in the child's Individualized Education Program (IEP). School nurse services are services provided by a qualified school nurse. School health services are services that may be provided by either a qualified school nurse or other qualified person" (34 CFR § 300.34(c)(15)). This "other qualified person" may be a speech-language pathologist (Power-deFur & Alley, 2008).

Implications of Case Law

IDEA provides significant protections for children and parents, including the right to dispute the decisions or actions of the district. Most disputes are resolved through discussion and mediation at the district level. However, some disputes may result in administrative hearings at the state level, often termed a "due process hearing." After exhausting administrative remedies, the losing party in the due process hearing may appeal to either state or federal court (Klare, 1997). As is common in special education, case law, the decisions of the administrative and court hearings, frequently interpret or clarify the statute or regulations. Special education personnel and school attorneys generally consider case law when refining local policies and procedures.

The following is a brief discussion of case law that has implications for serving children with feeding and swallowing issues in schools. It should be noted that this section is not considered to be a legal review or to provide legal advice. Districts are strongly advised to consult with their school board attorney for advice.

Two disputes that were resolved by the U.S. Supreme Court provide direction to schools in addressing their responsibilities with respect to health services. These cases are generally referred to as Tatro (*Irving Independent School District v. Tatro* [1984]) and Garrett (*Cedar Rapids Community School District v. Garrett F.* [1999]) (Power-deFur, 2009; Power-deFur & Alley, 2008). In both cases, children with severe physical disabilities required health-related services to participate in school. The position of the school districts was that the services were "medical services" and as such, were not part of the district's responsibility. The court decisions in these two cases clarified that the only permitted exclusion is for those medical services that must be provided by a physician, and that the services in question could, in fact, be rendered by non-physicians in the school setting. Ultimately, failure to provide the service could result in the child's inability to participate in the education program (Power-deFur, 2009; Power-deFur & Alley, 2008; Zirkel, 2005).

In the Tatro case, the U.S. Supreme Court ruled that clean, intermittent catheritization was not a "medical service," required only for diagnosis or evaluation, but a "school health service," defined as a service "provided by a qualified school nurse or other qualified person." This decision lends support to the notion that children with health care needs may also receive services to meet their day-to-day health needs. Fifteen years later, the U.S. Supreme Court ruled in the Garrett case that if related services are critical to the continual enrollment of an eligible child with a disability, then those services must be provided, as long as they are not purely medical in nature (Power-deFur & Alley, 2008). This case established the assumption that students with health care needs will attend school, just like their peers without health needs. Districts are responsible for ensuring that students receive the necessary health care services while they are attending school, thereby assuring their access to FAPE (National Association of School Nurses, 2013). This case further established that any noneducational service might also be a required service if it is deemed critical in keeping the child in school during the day. As such, this case makes provision for the evaluation and treatment of feeding and swallowing disorders.

The impact of the Garrett case may be seen in a review of state due process hearings since that time. In a New Mexico case in 2003, a state hearing officer found that "a service that enables a handicapped child to remain at school during the day is an important means of providing the child with the meaningful access to education that Congress envisioned" (New Mexico Department of Education, 103 LRP, 57798, SEA NM 2003). Further, the hearing officer identified that in order to remain in school, the student needed "access to foods that comply with the mechanical soft diet prescribed, . . . upright positioning during and after eating, thickening of all liquids . . . and careful monitoring for signs of reflux or aspiration" (New Mexico Department of Education, 103 LRP, 57798, SEA NM 2003). The hearing officer additionally concluded that provision of a "mechanical soft diet is a major factor in assuring adequate school health services." In a 2004 New Hampshire case, a state-level hearing officer concluded that the district denied the provision of a free and appropriate public education to a student with multiple disabilities who also had swallowing problems. Of note to this article, however, is the student's silent aspiration and consequent health problems. The district ignored the child's safety in its failure to address the diet and feeding recommendations found in the medical records. Medical evidence included the findings that the student exhibited a "severely weak pharyngeal swallow along with severe oral motor dysfunction" (Contoocook Valley School District, 41 IDELR 45, SEA NH 2004). The evidence was cited in the conclusion that inadequate feeding practices by the district "appear to have led to two hospital admissions for aspiration pneumonia" (Contoocock Valley School District, 41 IDELR 45, SEA NH 2004).

In Arkansas in 2012, a hearing officer identified the importance of having a detailed individualized health care plan and an emergency plan (Benton Sch. Dist., 113 LRP 17149; SEA AR 2012). In this situation, the detailed planning by the school district regarding the child's health care needs was important in resolution of the case. In Louisiana, (*Robertson v. E. Baton Rouge Parish Sch. Bd., No. 2012 CA 2039, 2013 WL 3947124, at *1* [La. Ct. App. July 29, 2013]) the court found that a district's failure to supervise a nonverbal student with visual impairment and development delays while he was eating resulted in a severe choking episode that ultimately contributed to the student's death. In this situation, a substitute teacher was feeding the child and not following the procedures expressed in the IEP.

These cases suggest that school personnel should be particularly aware of the health issues associated with swallowing and feeding. These issues, if not addressed in the form of a written protocol that clearly defines those strategies that are essential for maintaining student safety during feeding and swallowing, may further compromise the child's ability to attend and participate in school, thus limiting his or her ability to benefit from special education. School personnel are reminded to review case law and its implication, in consultation with appropriate legal counsel for the district.

Applying Special Education Policies and Procedures to Children With Dysphagia

Consider the two children discussed in the opening of this chapter. Both children were found to be eligible for special education; the team determined that the each child had a disability under IDEA that had an adverse effect on their education. These students are illustrative of the student for whom the speech-language impairment is a secondary disability. Although the disability could be speech-language impairment as the primary disability, it is more likely that speech-language impairment would be a secondary disability (e.g., secondary to a primary disability of orthopedic impairment, other health impairment, multiple disabilities, or intellectual disability). Approximately one-half of the children with disabilities who are served by speech-language pathologists have speech-language impairment as a secondary disability or related services, with a different primary disability (Power-deFur, 2011). For most of the children served with dysphagia, swallowing is one of many disorders that require services, and speech-language pathology services would logically be required.

As O'Toole stated (2000), the federal disability category that may be most appropriate to use with children with feeding and swallowing problems is "other health impairment." IDEA defines "other health impairment as "having limited strength, vitality, or alertness, including a heightened alertness to environmental stimuli, that results in limited alertness with respect to the educational environment, that (i) is due to chronic or acute health problems such as a heart condition, tuberculosis, rheumatic fever, nephritis, arthritis, asthma, sickle cell anemia, hemophilia, epilepsy, lead poisoning, leukemia, attention deficit disorder or attention deficit hyperactivity disorder, and diabetes; and (ii) adversely affects a child's educational performance" (IDEIA 34 CFR 34 CFR § 300.8(c)(9)). Although the definition's list of health conditions does not specifically include dysphagia, the definition is not a comprehensive list and allows for other health conditions that limit strength, vitality, or alertness. The category of "other health impairment" enables school districts to focus on the child's health care needs that must be attended to in order for children to stay in school. Obara (2011) identified that poor nutrition has an adverse effect on academic performance and that hunger has been associated with behavioral problems. Obara (2011) posits that improved nutritional state can lead to decreased school absenteeism for nutrition-related disorders, improved attention span, and increased energy levels. As seen in the later discussion of case law, these health needs may include focus on attendance because children will not have an educational benefit if their health needs prevent attendance at school. Due to the increased likelihood of swallowing-related aspiration in specific conditions, including cerebral palsy and traumatic brain injury (Miller, 2011), there is an increased likelihood that attendance may be impaired by the presence of a swallowing problem that is untreated and results in aspiration. Miller (2011) points out that children who have significant neurological impairment have higher possibility of silent aspiration.

After determination that the child with swallowing and feeding problems has a disability, the eligibility team then identifies whether there is an adverse educational impact of the disability. The team would keep in mind the principles of case law, specifically the Tatro and Garrett cases, by considering how the need for swallowing and feeding services relate to the child's ability to be in school to receive FAPE. Failure to provide swallowing and feeding services at school has the potential to deny the child the ability to remain in school. Because the school day generally includes the lunch meal, and often the breakfast meal, the child with dysphagia has the same rights as other students to receive nutrition safely at school.

The next criterion of the eligibility decision is whether the child needs special education and related services. As dysphagia services are not regarded as specially designed instruction, they are more likely to be identified as a related service, potentially as a speech-language service or a school health service. Although dysphagia intervention is clearly within the scope of practice of speech-language pathologists, a variety of school personnel are involved in the child's health, including the school nurse and school nutrition specialists; therefore, it may be more appropriate to consider it a school health service. The team would not exclude services to address dysphagia from the child's IEP under the contention that it is a medical service because persons who are not physicians may provide swallowing and feeding services.

Following determination of eligibility, the team will develop the child's IEP. This includes the child's present level of academic achievement and functional performance (PLAAFP), goals and objectives, and services. The PLAAFP could include a discussion of the child's feeding and swallowing needs. A goal addressing swallowing to ensure safety could be developed followed by identification of services designed to provide for safe feeding and swallowing. The goals and services will vary from child to child, based on the each child's unique needs. Some may focus on all services provided by school personnel whereas others may focus on the child's development of independent skills.

Schools have a legal responsibility to take reasonable steps to prevent students from foreseeable injury (Daggett, 2013). As districts cannot assume that a nurse will be present at all times, it is important that specific procedures be in place to handle emergencies. Many districts follow the standard care of practice of the nursing profession and develop an individual health care plan for the child. Such a plan typically includes a description of the child's medical history and current status, health care needs, medication, feeding and nutritional needs, staff training, and emergency procedures, as well as specific procedures required to address the child's health care needs (Lowman & Murphy, 1999; National Association of School Nurses, 2015). The health care plan may be separate from the IEP, referred to in the IEP, or incorporated into the IEP.

The National Association of School Nurses (NASN) (2015 highlights the importance of an "individualized healthcare plan (IHP)" for students who have health care needs that may affect the student's safety, school attendance, and academic performance. NASN identifies the development of the health care plan as the responsibility of the nurse, based on the standards of care established in the nurse practice acts within the state. The individualized health care plan is the foundation for student health interventions and should clarify the interventions, safe and appropriate delegation of care, and methods for review and evaluation of the plan. NASN identifies that the plan is a data source for multiple functions, including reimbursement and legal evidence. The plan may be incorporated into the child's IEP or be a stand-alone document that may be referred to in the IEP.

There are some children for whom feeding and swallowing issues are behavioral in nature. IDEA has provisions to address behavioral problems that interfere with the child's academic program or those of others. School personnel, including the speech-language pathologist, should work with behavioral specialists in the schools to evaluate the behavioral issues and assist in developing a behavioral intervention plan, as appropriate. Behaviorally based feeding issues should be addressed in accordance with these long-established IDEA procedures.

Collaboration with physicians is an important component of working with children with dysphagia in schools. In terms of determination of eligibility and IEP services, IDEA directs that schools must consider the reports of other professionals, but the decision remains with the eligibility and/or IEP team(s). Therefore, physician orders related to educational concerns (e.g., academic instruction, amount of services) should be considered by the eligibility and IEP teams, but the teams are not required to include the information from the orders. The final determination regarding eligibility and services is the role of the school-based teams, not the physician.

However, the physician is a valuable team member whose input is important in ensuring the child's healthy attendance at school. Districts have a long history of receiving and following physician's orders regarding medication, injuries, and medically related absences, as these clearly represent the intersection between the medical and educational communities. Districts collaborate with physicians to ensure they are attending to physician's orders related to medication, nutrition, and diet to ensure the child's ability to be safely fed at school. The school nurse is a valuable member of the child's dysphagia team, frequently the primary point of contact with the child's physician.

School Nutrition

The Child Nutrition and Women, Infants, and Children (WIC) Reauthorization Act of 2004 (P.L. 108-265 Section 204) mandates that all school districts participating in the National School Lunch

Program adopt and implement a local wellness policy (Castillo et al., 2010). This policy includes nutrition guidelines for school meals and all foods available on school campus, which would include the meals for students with dysphagia who require a different meal than the traditional school lunch. Further, this policy specifies a team approach to development of a local wellness policy, opening the door for the speech-language pathologists' engagement with school nutrition specialists in addressing the dietary and nutrition needs of children with dysphagia. It is the position of the American Dietetic Association (2010) that nutrition services provided by registered dieticians are essential components of comprehensive care for all people with developmental disabilities and special health care populations.

The U.S. Department of Agriculture promulgates regulations regarding school food service operations. These regulations address the needs of students with a disability, requiring schools to make substitutions in lunches and after school snacks for students considered to have a disability. Further, these are to be provided at no extra cost for children with special needs. (American Dietetic Association, 2010; Obara, 2011). Such a diet change must be supported by a written order from a recognized medical authority (generally a physician, physician's assistant, or nurse practitioner, as specified by each state). This order includes the disability and how it impacts the diet, major life activities affected by the disability, and a list of appropriate food substitutions, dietary changes and/or meal modifications (Obara, 2011). Note that the identification of disability may vary for IDEA and for qualification for dietary changes.

Rehabilitation Act and Americans With Disabilities Act

Children with dysphagia and other specialized health needs also receive protection under Section 504 of the Rehabilitation Act of 1973, frequently known as "Section 504" (29 U.S.C. §701 et seq.) This law provides that no otherwise qualified individual shall, solely by reasons of his or her disability, be excluded from participation in, be denied benefits of, or be subject to discrimination under any program receiving federal financial assistance. Any program receiving federal financial assistance, including public schools, is bound by the requirements of this statute (United States Department of Education, 2005). Section 504 defines a "person with a disability" as any person who "has a physical or mental impairment which substantially limits one or more of life's major activities" (29 U.S.C. §706(8)(B)). Dysphagia is certainly a physical impairment that limits one of life's major activities: eating and drinking (U.S. Department of Education, 2012). As such, children with dysphagia are likely to be eligible for services under Section 504. Castillo et al. report that Section 504 requires school nutrition programs to accommodate children with disabilities who have a diet prescription (2010). However, Section 504 does not include funding for programs. The consequence of this is that many school districts will find children with disabilities, including students with feeding and swallowing disorders, to be eligible under IDEA rather than Section 504. This practice, however, does not negate the value of Section 504 as a civil rights law that can protect persons with dysphagia from discrimination.

The Americans with Disabilities Act is another federal law that protects the rights of persons with disabilities (U.S. DOE, 1990). Established in 1990, this is a national mandate to address discrimination in all sectors, including education, employment, transportation, public accommodations, and telecommunications (Office for Civil Rights, n.d.a, n.d.b). School districts' obligations under ADA and Section 504 are comparable, as ADA references Section 504 in the area of education (Klare, 1997).

Medicaid

In 1988, Congress authorized Medicaid as a source of funding for certain services provided to children receiving special education. This action made it acceptable for schools to access Medicaid funds for services provided to a child eligible for Medicaid that is covered by the state Medicaid policy and provided by Medicaid-qualified school personnel (American Speech-Language-Hearing Association, 2004; Herz, 2006; Kander, 2010). IDEA specified that, contrary to the Medicaid policy that Medicaid is the payer of last resort; the financial responsibility of Medicaid must precede the financial responsibility of the local and state education agencies (Herz, 2006). Medicaid is a federal-state program, with funding from both federal and state governments. States must adhere to all federal requirements, yet they have authority to establish parameters of each state's program. As a result, specific Medicaid requirements regarding services, personnel, and eligibility vary from state to state.

The Medicaid program for children requires identification of children in need of health services and the provision of services to screen, diagnose, and treat such children. Most children requiring dysphagia services will be eligible for Medicaid due to their complex medical needs. Medicaid's health services include speech-language pathology, audiology, occupational therapy, physical therapy, and nursing services (American Speech-Language-Hearing Association, 2004). Swallowing and feeding services may be reimbursable under Medicaid under either or both speech-language pathology and nursing services. Medicaid rules do not specify how Medicaid funds received by school districts may be used. Ideally, funds generated by serving children with dysphagia will be returned to the special education program.

Title XIX of the Social Security Act funds Medicaid, which provides medical services for individuals and families with low income. Medicaid may pay for services such as special dietary supplements, eating devices, and nutritional consultation, when deemed medically necessary (American Dietetic Association, 2010).

State Guidance

The responsibility for implementation of IDEA within the state is delegated by IDEA to the State Education Agencies (SEA), the state departments of education. Some SEAs have speech-language consultants who work collaboratively with other special education professionals to provide direction regarding services for children with swallowing disorders in schools. For example, the SEAs in North Carolina and Virginia both address dysphagia in their guidelines for speech-language services in schools (North Carolina Department of Public Instruction, 2006;

Virginia Department of Education, 2011). Further, SEAs manage the school nutrition programs, providing direction regarding school food programs and nutrition and providing training and technical assistance to districts throughout their states. A third resource at the state level is the school health/nurse specialists at the state education agency and/or the state departments of health. These professionals and their programs provide guidance regarding design and implementation of school health plans. School-based teams serving children with dysphagia are wise to review guidance documents from their state education and health departments and contact consultants at either state agency for direction.

Ethical Issues

As professionals, speech-language pathologists are bound by the duty to care for their clients, a duty that places certain responsibilities on the profession. These duties include meeting the expected requirements of the law (e.g., IDEA) and regulations, of the scope of practice for the profession, and of evidence-based practices. Furthermore, speech-language pathologists strive to provide the best quality care for their clients and to protect them from harm. Huffman and Owre (2008) highlight that ethical issues related to serving children with dysphagia can arise from a variety of circumstances, which can include operating procedures, legal/regulatory and reimbursement requirements, and employer expectations.

Speech-language pathologists who are certified by the American Speech-Language-Hearing Association (ASHA) and/or are members of ASHA are bound by the ASHA Code of Ethics (American Speech-Language-Hearing Association, 2010a). The Code of Ethics centers around four principles: welfare of the client, achieve and maintain the highest levels of competence, honor responsibility to the public, and honor responsibility to the professions. The principles of ethics are considered to be both aspirational and inspirational. Each of these principles is elucidated by a number of rules of ethics, statements of minimally acceptable professional conduct or of prohibitions. Together, the principles and rules are designed as affirmative obligations for professionals, regardless of professional setting or situation.

Whereas all four principles are relevant to all aspects of the practice of speech-language pathology, the first two have clear connection to this chapter. Principle I, the welfare of the person served, includes such rules as providing services competently; using every resource, including referral when appropriate; maintaining appropriate documentation and not discriminating. Principle II, professional competence, includes rules related to providing services only when qualified and not permitting persons to provide services beyond their competence.

Professional preparation and competence are critical in all aspects of the field of speech-language pathology and no less so for serving children with swallowing and feeding disorders (Power-deFur, 2000). Two recent studies have investigated school speech-language pathologists' levels of confidence in providing dysphagia services in schools. Studies by O'Donoghue and Dean-Claytor (2008) and Hutchins, Gerety, and Mulligan (2011) found that a number of school-based speech-language pathologists had low levels of confidence in their ability to provide dysphagia services. O'Donoghue and Dean-Claytor (2008) found that some speech-language pathologists who had some training in the provision of dysphagia services felt less confident than those who did not have any training. They conjectured that this might be because the speech-language pathologist with some training recognized the magnitude of the responsibility associated with providing services. In contrast, Hutchins et al. (2011) found a positive relationship, indicating that speech-language pathologists who had training had greater confidence in their ability to provide skilled service. Both studies highlight the ethical obligation school-based speech-language pathologists have to gain appropriate education and training to competently serve children with feeding and swallowing issues in schools.

In light of the duty to provide no harm to the client, such professional development needs to be sufficient in order to gain competence. Failure to attain this competency can result in (i) failure to provide services to the student; and (ii) provision of services by personnel who do not have adequate knowledge to attend to the child's safety and swallowing needs. The school-based speech-language pathologist who is aware of the need to serve one or more children with dysphagia will need to ensure the welfare of the client is maintained. The speech-language pathologist will find it valuable to reflect on the situation with the following questions:

- Do I have the skills to work with children with swallowing and feeding issues? If not, how can I acquire those skills? If I am working to acquire these skills, can I master them soon enough to meet the child's needs in a manner that does no harm? Is it more appropriate to make a referral to another speech-language pathologist and/or a swallowing and feeding team?
- Am I maintaining appropriate documentation of services for these children, including documentation of efforts to ensure the children's safety?
- Are non-skilled personnel providing swallowing and feeding services to the child during mealtime or snack time? Are these persons appropriately trained to provide this service safely? If not, what is my obligation to ensure they are appropriately trained?

Huffman and Owre (2008) identify a variety of ethically appropriate responses a school-based speech-language pathologist may take related to his or her competence. Attainment of competency is clearly the most important step. However, Huffman and Owre also highlight the importance of alerting school administration regarding the limitations in competency. They further emphasize that it would be ethically questionable to provide services without adequate knowledge and skills or to avoid any involvement, thereby denying the child services.

School-based speech-language pathologists may feel they are confronted with an ethical dilemma, such as those presented in the opening paragraph of this chapter. Two children were described that show signs and symptoms of dysphagia, yet the children's feeding and swallowing needs were not being addressed in accordance with best practices and the welfare of the children. When faced with concerns related to a child's safety, disagreement with team members and/or the administration, and legal expectations, the speech-language pathologist may find it valuable to apply an ethical decision-making model to achieve resolution. Such an approach would involve 5 steps:

1. Gather the facts of the situation. Review the child's record to gather information from the IEP, 504 plan, and/or individual health care plan. Review medical records on file. Talk with teachers and school administrators regarding the children's behavior, absenteeism, interventions used at school, and gather information from the parent/guardian.

2. Determine if this is a legal and/or ethical situation. A review of the information in this chapter will assist in sorting out any legal/regulatory requirements. In addition, the speech-language pathologist will want to review state policy documents and local district policies and procedures. A review of the ASHA Code of Ethics and ASHA documents related to ethics will elucidate any ethical situations.

3. Consult with others. The speech-language pathologist may find it valuable to contact the following: the speech-language specialist at the state education agency, the Medicaid specialist at the state education and/or medical agency, and/or staff at the American Speech-Language-Hearing Association who work in school and health services. In addition, consultation with other speech-language pathologists in the district and in neighboring districts will be valuable. The speech-language pathologist will also want to consult with the school nurse, the school nutrition director, and the special education administrator.

4. Brainstorm actions. These could include such actions as: creation of an individualized health care plan, request consultation from another speech-language pathologist with expertise, referral to another speech-language pathologist in the district or outside of the district.

5. Select action and act. The speech-language pathologist should select an action that results in resolution of the situation. Although it is possible that the speech-language pathologist may find that errors have been made

in the past, it is often best to move toward a solution that begins afresh, providing for the welfare of the child and meeting the legal and ethical obligations of the professionals and the district.

As with all decisions, it is important to establish a time frame for implementation and for review of the results. Frequently, there is no single "right" response, highlighting the need to reflect upon the action to determine if the ethical situation is being resolved. If this review suggests that the ethical issues remain, then steps three through five should be repeated.

Best Practice

The preceding review of special education, disability, and Medicaid requirements informs best practice in the provision of services to children with swallowing and feeding disorders. The following recommendations are offered to school-based speech-language pathologists and their swallowing and feeding team members to facilitate compliance with legal requirements, to minimize liability and ethical challenges, and, most importantly, to assure that students' needs are met.

1. School districts should identify if their state education agency has regulations, policies, or guidance documents related to serving children with dysphagia and their nutrition and secure such documents or if the SEA provides training and technical assistance. Districts should check with their state Medicaid and education agencies regarding specific children's eligibility for Medicaid in order to determine whether that state's Medicaid state plan covers dysphagia services in schools. School-based teams should review relevant documents and participate in training as a team. District personnel should advocate for policies, guidelines, and professional development as needed.
2. Speech-language pathologists should work as members of a team when serving children with dysphagia. In

addition to the speech-language pathologist, the team should include the parent(s), school nurse, the school nutrition specialist, teacher(s), parent(s), occupational and physical therapist(s), paraprofessionals, the child's primary medical provider, and the principal or other administrators. The speech-language pathologist will want to collaborate with the school nutrition specialist in identifying and securing diet modifications and with the school nurse in developing an individualized health care plan.

3. School districts should ensure that they have a cadre of personnel with appropriate training and competence to assess and intervene on behalf of children with swallowing and feeding disorders. The training should address the professional standards of practice of the professions to demonstrate that the speech-language pathologist and other members of the child's team are exercising a reasonable standard of care in his or her duties. Speech-language pathologists are instrumental personnel in planning and providing training that is individualized to the needs of each child with dysphagia. Participants in training would include, but not be limited to, the speech-language pathologist, special education teachers and paraprofessionals, occupational therapists, and school nurses and nursing assistants. Districts should be certain that any new personnel involved in feeding the child, including substitutes, be appropriately trained. Completion of training and demonstration of competency should be documented.

4. Speech-language pathologists should screen any child whose background suggests the presence of dysphagia. Diagnostic evaluations should be conducted for any student for whom the screening suggests the presence of dysphagia. The school nurse, principal, special education administration and other pertinent administrators should be informed promptly of the need for an evaluation. The assessment may be conducted as part of the child's evaluation for special education eligibility. The school speech-language pathologist may conduct this assessment or refer to and/or collaborate

with other speech-language pathologists. Due to the urgent health issues that may accompany dysphagia, the district should establish policy that allows for the immediate evaluation of a child's feeding and swallowing for safety purposes.

5. Medical records should be secured, especially records related to assessments (e.g., modified barium swallow studies) and medical orders related to diet and nutrition. Frequently, the child's physician will issue an order associated with the child's health care needs, including dysphagia. The school nurse typically is the team member who ensures that these physicians' orders are carried out. District personnel should be careful to consider all recommendations for diet or feeding that are provided by outside medical providers and engage those providers to ensure consistent planning to meet the child's swallowing and feeding issues. Swallowing and feeding teams should continue to monitor children's health and absenteeism to determine if there is any relationship between the child's swallowing and feeding issues and his or her absenteeism

6. Team members should maintain communication with outside medical providers (e.g., hospital-based speech-language pathologists, radiologists, and other physicians). The school speech-language pathologist should assume responsibility for communication with the hospital-based SLP and/or radiologist regarding the results of the modified barium swallow, as well as with any other speech-language pathologist who provides services to the child. The school nurse and school nutrition specialists may need to communicate with the child's physician to secure any needed physician's order they may need to provide services and/or modify the child's diet. Effective service delivery is built upon clear communication with outside medical personnel who serve the child.

7. As dysphagia is a health issue, the child's health needs can be addressed immediately. The child's dysphagia requires direct and immediate intervention and should not wait for determination of special education eligibility. School health services develop an individualized health

care plan (IHP) for children with health care needs as part of the standard of practice. District personnel should develop such a plan promptly whenever a child is identified who requires swallowing and feeding services while at school. The health care plan can be incorporated into the child's IEP or serve as a stand-alone document, depending on state and district policy. The health care plan should include a description of the child's medical history and current status, health care needs, medication, feeding and nutritional needs, transportation and restroom arrangements, and any specific procedures required to address the child's health care needs (National Association of School Nurses, 2013). Specific procedures related to swallowing and feeding should identify the roles and responsibilities of the speech-language pathologist, nurse, teacher(s), paraprofessional(s), and others working with the child. In addition, the health plan should address emergency procedures.

8. Districts should ensure that the IEP and any health care plan are adhered to for all children, including children with dysphagia. Each person working with the child on swallowing and feeding (including substitute personnel) should have a current copy. The IEP and/or health care plan should be reviewed and amended whenever there is evidence that there is a change in the child's feeding and swallowing status.

9. Swallowing and feeding teams should consider whether the child's behavior is associated with swallowing and feeding. The team should make a referral for a functional behavioral analysis to identify if there are underlying or associated behaviors that should be addressed. As the specialist in swallowing, the speech-language pathologist should be a participant in this analysis. The functional behavioral analysis may indicate the need for a behavioral intervention plan for feeding. Again, the speech-language pathologist should be part of the team developing the plan, to assure integration with the feeding and swallowing services identified on the IEP and/or health plan.

10. All district personnel working with the child should maintain adequate and appropriate documentation regarding the provision of services according to the IEP or IHP. A daily log of feeding activities could be used to document daily feeding activities. Response to any emergency situation, in accordance with the procedures established in the health plan, should be documented.

11. Due to the schools' responsibility for the safety and well-being of students during school hours on school property and during school-sponsored activities, schools should have written procedures and policies for managing first aid emergencies. Speech-language pathologists should work with other school personnel in reviewing these emergency protocols to ensure that they appropriately address swallowing and feeding issues, especially actions to be taken in the event a child aspirates. Sufficient school personnel qualified to perform cardiopulmonary resuscitation (CPR) should be available in all buildings. The districts' emergency protocols should include indicators for referral to outside medical providers.

Conclusion

School-based speech-language pathologists are wise to consider the legal and ethical issues associated with serving children with swallowing and feeding challenges who are in public schools. These children have a right to receive the swallowing and feeding services they need in a public school setting. A review of the statutes, regulations, and case law indicates that children needing dysphagia services are entitled to receive them in order to ensure their health, safety, and attendance, all of which are necessary in accessing a free appropriate public education. With the knowledge of these legal, regulatory, and ethical issues, school-based speech-language pathologists are better able to educate school administrators and advocate for and address the needs of children with dysphagia in schools. As a first step, districts will want to create an interdisciplinary swallowing and feeding

team and charge that team with responsible for creating policies and procedures, ensuring professional development for key
personnel working with these children, and the development
and adherence to emergency procedures. With these policies
and procedures in place, the team can confidently serve children
with swallowing and feeding disorders in schools.

References

American Dietetic Association. (2010). Position of the American Dietetic
Association: Providing nutrition services for people with develop-
mental disabilities and special health care needs. *Journal of the
American Dietetic Association, 110,* 296–307.
American Speech-Language-Hearing Association. (2004). *Medicaid
guidance for speech language pathology services: Addressing the
"under the direction of rule* [Technical report]. Rockville, MD: Author.
American Speech-Language-Hearing Association. (2007). *Scope of prac-
tice in speech language pathology.* Rockville, MD: Author.
American Speech-Language-Hearing Association. (2010a). *Code of ethics.*
Rockville, MD: Author.
American Speech-Language-Hearing Association. (2010b). *Roles and
responsibilities of speech-language pathologists in schools.* Rockville,
MD: Author.
American Speech-Language-Hearing Association. (2012). *2012 schools
survey.* Rockville, MD: Author.
Assistance to States for the Education of Children with Disabilities and
the Early Intervention Program for Infants and Toddlers with Dis-
abilities: Final Rule, 71 Fed. Reg. 46570 (2006).
Benton Sch. Dist., 113 LRP 17149 (SEA AR 2012).
Castillo, A., Carr, D., & Nettles, M. F. (2010). Best practices for serv-
ing students with special food and/or nutrition needs in school
nutrition programs. *School Nutrition Association, 34.* Retrieved
from https://schoolnutrition.org/5--News-and-Publications/4--The-
Journal-of-Child-Nutrition-and-Management/Fall-2010/Volume-34,
-Issue-2,-Fall-2010---Castillio;-Carr;-Nettles/
Cedar Rapids Community School District v. Garrett F, 526 U.S. 66 (1999).
Cerezo, C. S., Lobato, D. J., Pinkos, B., & LeLeiko, N. S. (2011). Diagnosis and treatment of pediatric feeding and swallowing disorders:
The team approach. *ICAN: Infant, Child, & Adolescent Nutrition, 3,*
321–323.

Contoocook Valley School District, 41 IDELR 45 (SEA NH 2004).
Daggett, L. M. (2013). Reasonable supervision in the city: Enhancing the safety of students with disabilities in urban (and other) schools. *Fordham Urban Law Journal, 41,* 501–556.
Education for all Handicapped Children Act (EAHCA), 20 U.S.C. § 1400 *et seq.* (1975).
Herz, E. J. (2006, March 9). *The link between Medicaid and the Individuals with Disabilities Education Act (IDEA): Recent history and current issues.* Washington, DC: Congressional Research Service.
Huffman, N. P., & Owre, D. W. (2008). Ethical issues in providing services in schools to children with swallowing and feeding disorders. *Language, Speech, and Hearing Services in Schools, 39,* 167–176.
Hutchins, T. L., Gerety, K. W., & Mulligan, M. (2011). Dysphagia management: A survey of school-based speech-language pathologists in Vermont. *Language, Speech, and Hearing Services in Schools, 42,* 194–206.
Individuals with Disabilities Education Improvement Act of 2004, 20 U.S.C. § 1400 et seq. (2004).
Individuals with Disabilities Education Improvement Act, 34 C.F.R. Part 104 (2006).
Irving Independent School District v. Tatro, 468 U.S. 883 (1984).
Kander, M. (2010, September). Medicaid reimbursement in schools. *ASHA Leader, 15,* 3–29.
Klare, K. (1997). Legal concerns. In L. A. Power-deFur & F. P. Orelove (Eds.), *Inclusive education: Practical implementation of the least restrictive environment* (pp. 43–62). Gaithersburg, MD: Aspen.
Lowman, D. K., & Murphy, S. M. (1999). *The educator's guide to feeding children with disabilities.* Baltimore, MD: Paul H. Brookes.
Miller, C. K. (2011). Aspiration and swallowing dysfunction in pediatric patients. *ICAN: Infant, Child & Adolescent Nutrition, 3,* 336–343.
National Association of School Nurses. (2013). *Position statement: Section 504 and Individuals with Disabilities Education Improvement Act–The role of the school nurse.* Retrieved from http://www.nasn.org/PolicyAdvocacy/PositionPapersandReports/NASNPositionStatements
National Association of School Nurses. (2015). *Position statement: Individualized healthcare plans: The role of the school nurse.* Retrieved August 31, 2014, from http://www.nasn.org/PolicyAdvocacy/PositionPapersandReports/NASNPositionStatements
New Mexico Department of Education, 103 LRP 57798 (SEA NM 2003).
North Carolina Department of Public Instruction. (2006). *North Carolina Guidelines for Speech-Language Pathology Services in Schools.* Raleigh, NC: Author.

Obara, M. (2011, Jan/Feb). Nutrition issues facing children with special health care needs in early intervention programs and at school. *Nutrition Focus for Children with Special Health Care Needs, 26*(1), 1–10.

O'Donoghue, C. R. & Dean-Claytor, A. D. (2008). Training and self-reported confidence for dysphagia management among speech-language pathologists in the schools. *Language, Speech, and Hearing Services in Schools, 39,* 192–198.

Office for Civil Rights. (n.d.a.) *Americans with Disabilities Act (ADA).* Retrieved August 29, 2014, from http://www.ed.gov/about/offices/list/ocr/docs/hq9805.html

Office for Civil Rights (n.d.b). *Questions and Answers on Disability Discrimination under Section 504 and Title II.* Retrieved August 29, 2014, from http://www.ed.gov/about/offices/list/ocr/qa-disability.html

O'Toole, T. J. (2000). Legal, ethical, and financial aspects of providing services to children with swallowing disorders in public schools. *Language, Speech, and Hearing Services in Schools, 31,* 56–61.

Power-deFur, L. (2000). Serving students with dysphagia in the schools? Educational preparation is essential! *Language, Speech, and Hearing Services in Schools, 31,* 76–78.

Power-deFur, L. (2009). Dysphagia services in schools: Applying special education requirements to a health service. *Perspectives on Swallowing and Swallowing Disorders, 18,* 86–90.

Power-deFur, L. (2011, April). When is a child with speech-language impairment a child with a disability? Special education eligibility criteria. *ASHA Leader, 16,* 12–15.

Power-deFur, L., & Alley, N. S. N. (2008). Legal and financial issues associated with providing services in schools to children with swallowing and feeding disorders. *Language, Speech, and Hearing Services in Schools, 39,* 160–166.

Rehabilitation Act of 1973, as amended, 29 U.S.C. §794 (1973).

Robertson v. E. Baton Rouge Parish Sch. Bd., No. 2012 CA 2039, 2013 WL 3947124, at *1 (La. Ct. App. July 29, 2013).

U. S. Department of Education. (1990). *Americans with Disabilities Act (ADA).* Retrieved August 13, 2014, from http://www.ed.gov/about/offices/list/ocr/docs/hq9805.html

U. S. Department of Education. (2012). *Questions and answers on disability discrimination under Section 504 and Title III.* Retrieved August 13, 2014, from http://www.ed.gov/about/offices/list/ocr/qa-disability.html

U. S. Department of Education, Office of Special Education and Rehabilitative Services, Office of Special Education Programs. (2005). *25th Annual (2003) Report to Congress on the Implementation of the Individuals with Disabilities Education Act* (Vol. 2). Washington, DC: Author.

Virginia Department of Education. (2011). *Speech language pathology services in schools: Guidelines for best practice.* Richmond, VA: Author.

Zirkel, P. (2005). A primer on special education law. *Teaching Exceptional Children, 38*(1), 62–63.

3

A Time-Tested Procedure for Addressing Swallowing and Feeding in the School Setting

Emily M. Homer

Addressing Swallowing and Feeding in the Schools: Making It Work!

Once a school system has agreed to adopt a procedure for addressing swallowing and feeding, it will be necessary to design a procedure that will fit within the rules and regulations of the school district and the state. When designing an interdisciplinary swallowing and feeding team procedure, each system will need to mold it to fit within these parameters. There is not one procedure that will work for every system. The procedure that follows has the essential components that may be adapted to almost any school district. All procedures should include specific steps on how to proceed when a swallowing and feeding disorder is suspected, a description of the suggested roles and responsibilities of the team of professionals, proper training on all levels within the school system, administrative support as well as financial support in terms of instrumental diagnostics, and therapeutic intervention. Careful preparation of a comprehensive swallowing and feeding procedure will facilitate the task of getting a district to adopt the procedure (Homer, Bickerton, Hill, Parham, & Taylor, 2000).

In addition to a well-designed procedure, it is essential that a team approach be utilized when addressing swallowing and feeding disorders. This chapter discusses working as a team; defining suggested roles and responsibilities of school based team members as well as presenting a procedure that can be adapted and utilized in other districts. Swallowing and feeding disorders always have a safety component that is extremely important.

Essential Component: Team Approach to Swallowing and Feeding in the Schools

Introduction to Working as a Team

Professionals working in the school setting are extremely familiar with the team approach. Collaborative teaming today drives school systems and those who work in special education are members of a variety of teams. Some of the teams that are common in school districts are grade level teams, student assistance teams, school improvement teams, 504 teams, positive behavior teams, and IEP teams. Teaming in the public schools has proven to be an effective tool in providing the best services to students. Regardless of the setting, swallowing and feeding is almost always addressed by a team of professionals. A true interdisciplinary approach involves each member of the group sharing the philosophy for diagnosis and treatment in addition to being willing and able to work with other team members within the group (Arvedson & Brodsky, 2002). It is essential that the team approach be done well with respect for each professional's field. To work effectively as a team, each team member must be willing to

- be aware of each person's role;
- share information;

- realize personal and professional limitations in relation to swallowing and feeding;
- be open to suggestions and to problem solving; and
- have open communication with team members.

Student Profile: Working as a Team

Katie is a high school student with cerebral palsy who has been followed by the swallowing and feeding team for years. When Katie moved on to the high school, her new case manager worked with the classroom teacher, OT, and nurse to establish a safe swallowing and feeding plan. The following year, a new OT was assigned to the high school. The SLP, the case manager, met with the classroom teacher and updated the plan and included some food precautions (a list of foods that were risky for the student to eat at school). The SLP did not consult with the new OT or the parent but went ahead and wrote the plan. The new OT assigned to the school knew Katie and her parents well through the years and did not agree with the extent of the restrictions. The OT went directly to the parents and then the teacher and shared with them her disagreement with the plan. The OT went ahead and revised the swallowing and feeding plan without consulting with the SLP. As a result, parents were very upset, the classroom teacher was torn between two professionals and team members, and the entire process was compromised.

Both the SLP (case manager) and the OT were at fault. The SLP was operating on her own and not as a team member, much less as a case manager. She should have consulted with the new OT, shared the potential changes with the parents, and worked with the classroom teacher. The OT was also not operating as a team member. With her initial concern, she should have met with the SLP to talk about her knowledge of the child, her concerns about the strict precautions, and encourage the team to meet with the parents. Together they should have had a meeting to discuss the student's safety issues and to come to a consensus as to what Katie's diet should look like at school. Many problems can occur when a team does not work together.

There are two interdisciplinary teams that are responsible for the identification and treatment of students in school systems, the school-based team and the medical team. The school-based team is comprised of professionals who in most cases are already employed by the school district. Listed below are some common school swallowing and feeding team members:

• Speech-language pathologist
• Occupational therapist
• School nurse
• Physical therapist
• Parents/guardians
• Special education teacher
• Regular education teacher
• Paraprofessional/classroom assistant
• School administrator
• Social worker
• Cafeteria manager/workers

Each listed team member has an important role to play in ensuring that children are safe at school and receive adequate nutrition and hydration.

There are times in the school system, when addressing swallowing and feeding, where it is necessary to work with a student's physician(s). This is significantly more difficult in the school setting and requires the cooperation of the parents/guardians. In most cases, in order to speak to a physician, it is necessary to have a signed release of information from the parents/guardians. It is recommended that these be signed at the IEP meeting where the student's swallowing and feeding concerns are initially discussed. This will facilitate the process of sharing and receiving information from physicians. When the team has a concern that requires information from the student's physician, the first step would be to meet with or talk to the student's parents/guardians about the concern and then follow up with the physician. The medical-based team frequently consists of the following:

• Student's primary care physician, gastroenterologist, pulmonologist, neurologist, or other physician.

- Hospital-based SLP
- Radiologist
- Registered dietician

It may be important to contact a physician under the following circumstances:

- When you have a serious concern about the student's health status
- To request a script for a Modified Barium Swallow Study/ Videofluoroscopic Swallow Study or Fiberoptic Endoscopic Examination
- To request a change in diet orders for a modified cafeteria diet. If the student's swallowing and feeding plan indicates that the food be altered prior to being put on the student's cafeteria tray, such as puree, then it would be necessary to receive a written script to modify the school lunch
- When you are concerned about a child's nutritional intake
- To get a more thorough medical history
- To clarify a script written by the doctor for a specific diet order or therapeutic intervention

It is essential that conversations with physicians be documented and placed in the student's special education folder.

Making Time for Team Collaboration

In school districts around the country, time remains one of the greatest challenges for therapists and nurses. High caseloads/ workloads, increasing regular education responsibilities and essential documentation result in SLPs, OTs, and nurses struggling to find time to meet all of the demands. Team collaboration is one of the most difficult tasks to accomplish due to team members having different schedules and demands. However, team collaboration is extremely important in diagnosing and treating swallowing and feeding in the schools. Team members will need to be creative in finding ways to discuss the student's needs. The core team of the speech pathologist, occupational therapist, and the school nurse will need to discuss the student's signs and symptoms and design a swallowing and feeding plan that addresses the student's issues and allows for safe feeding at school. Some suggestions for team collaboration are:

- Core team members include swallowing and feeding team collaboration on their weekly schedule. This could be as little as 15 to 20 minutes per week and could be as needed. If collaboration is not needed one week then there is extra time for other duties.
- E-mail correspondence regarding the student's needs. There should be caution when discussing a student in an e-mail. All e-mail discussions should be professional and focus only on a student's skills and abilities. While it can be a good tool for collaboration, it is important that school-based personnel realize that e-mails at any time can be requested by parents and therefore should always be a professional communication.
- Case manager is responsible for compiling information provided by the core team members as well as the teachers and parents/guardians, and distributing the information to other team members when indicated.

Case Manager System for Team and Case Management

Whenever there is a procedure that must be followed, team members that need to collaborate, and documentation that is required, there must be someone designated to oversee the process. It is recommended that districts use a case manager system to ensure that the procedure is being followed correctly, that team members are informed, and that the process is documented.

Each student that is being followed by the swallowing and feeding team should be assigned a case manager. The case manager should be the team member who is most knowledgeable about the disorder and the student. In many cases, the SLP assumes this role. If a district does not have a trained SLP or OT then they will need to investigate other ways to manage swallowing and feeding in the schools. Solutions when a district does not have trained therapists are covered in Chapter 9.

It is suggested that a case manager be assigned to each school in the district at the beginning of each school year, regardless of whether or not there are any students identified with swallowing and feeding concerns. This ensures that, when a student at each school is identified as having a swallowing and feeding disorder, there is a professional ready to coordinate and address the issues. The case manager is responsible for the following:

- Ensuring that the procedure is followed with fidelity
- Ensuring that all efforts are properly documented and kept in a student's file
- Notifying team members when changes in a student's swallowing and feeding skills occur
- Coordinating the student's swallowing and feeding services
- Providing information on a regular basis to the district swallowing and feeding administrator

The case manager is the person responsible for completing the paperwork associated with swallowing and feeding. They also work closely with teachers and parents to monitor changes in the student's skills at mealtimes. For example, if a student appears to be doing fine when eating lunch but then appears to struggle after, then the case manager may contact the team nurse to investigate gastroesophageal reflux. In this case, a medical referral may be needed and the school nurse would need to evaluate the student prior to recommending that the parent pursue a medical evaluation. It is extremely important that the person assigned as case manager have a broad knowledge of the various complications that may occur in students with swallowing and feeding disorders.

Essential Component: Defined Roles and Responsibility of Swallowing and Feeding Team Members

Every team member has a role to perform when addressing swallowing and feeding in the school setting. While each team member brings to the team effort-specific knowledge and skills in their respective disciplines, all team members are responsible for the following at their school sites:

- Referring a student to the swallowing and feeding team when they observe signs or symptoms of a swallowing or feeding disorder
- Monitoring students who are being followed by the team
- Overseeing the safety and well-being of students with swallowing and feeding disorders

An interdisciplinary team approach entails each member of a group of professionals providing their own specific area of expertise.

Typical Team Role: Speech-Language Pathologists

The speech-language pathologist in the school setting has a primary responsibility in the area of swallowing and feeding. The SLP is often the professional in the school with the most training and experience with swallowing and feeding. Many SLPs have extensive training at the graduate school level in the identification and treatment of dysphagia in children and adults. This training can be the foundation for management in the school setting. Typically the SLP may be responsible for the following:

- Referring students who show signs and symptoms of swallowing and feeding disorders
- Identifying students who are at risk by coordinating and conducting an interdisciplinary observation
- Functioning as the swallowing and feeding case manager for students on their caseload
- Coordinating assessment and treatment
- Participating in the instrumental examinations such as the MBSS/VFSS and/or FEES by attending the study with the student and parents/guardians.
- Attending IEP meetings as a member of the IEP committee for students with swallowing and feeding disorders
- Writing swallowing and feeding plans, with the input of other team members

- Training teachers and classroom staff on the implementation of the swallowing and feeding team
- Treating oral and pharyngeal phase dysphagia when indicated including oral awareness, texture and taste progression, chewing, and so on
- Consulting, and monitoring esophageal phase with medical referral when indicated
- Responding to issues and concerns regarding the student's swallowing and feeding disorder
- Attending ongoing professional development on swallowing and feeding disorders

Typical Team Role: Parent/Guardian

The parents/guardians are extremely important when addressing swallowing and feeding in the schools and play an essential role in the interdisciplinary team approach. Parents/guardians are the experts when it comes to knowing and caring for their child. Their experience has often taught them effective ways of dealing with their children's unique swallowing and feeding issues. The role of the parent on the swallowing and feeding team is often to:

- Share knowledge of their child's feeding habits, food preferences, and mealtime environment
- Provide medical information, including medications and history, to the school-based team as well as to provide releases for school staff and medical providers to collaborate
- Share their cultural view regarding mealtimes, foods, and eating habits with the school-based team
- Report to the case manager any changes in the child's swallowing and feeding skills and/or medical status
- Implement the swallowing and feeding goals at home

Typical Team Role: Occupational Therapist

Occupational therapists play an important role in the identification and treatment of swallowing and feeding disorders in the

---

Student Profile: Parent Cooperation

Hayden was an elementary student with hydroencephaly, an intact midbrain, and the remainder of her brain poorly developed. She was fed by PEG tube when the school swallowing and feeding team was initially established but was also being fed a slightly modified regular diet. Hayden had no chewing ability and a severely delayed swallow. The school team had serious concerns that Hayden would choke at school as well as aspirate. Hayden's parents were not receptive to a modified diet or to a referral for an MBSS. The school team told the mother that because of the safety risks of feeding Hayden at school that they must have clearance from her physician and doctor orders for an MBSS.

Mother took Hayden to the study but did not inform the school team of the day or time and therefore there was not a representative from the district at the study. At a follow-up meeting, the parent stated that the swallow study indicated that she was safe for an oral regular diet. She refused to share the report with the school team. The school team consulted with their legal team and it was determined that the district needed the medical report in order to feed Hayden orally at school. The district could provide the tube feedings at school. Hayden's mother decided not to share the MBSS report with the school team (which the team later found out recommended non per os (NPO or nothing by mouth). The mother continued to demand oral feeding and, as a result, chose to home school Hayden. Several years later, Hayden was reenrolled in the district where the mother was cooperative with the school team in establishing a swallowing and feeding plan that was NPO with no oral feeding at all. Hayden continues to do well.

---

school setting. They, along with the SLP and school nurse, make up the core team of professionals responsible for swallowing and feeding disorders. The OT brings extensive knowledge to the areas of feeding therapy, sensory integration, positioning, and adaptive equipment. The OT may be responsible for the following:

- Referring students who exhibit signs and symptoms of swallowing and feeding disorders
- Conducting the interdisciplinary observation along with the SLP, nurse, classroom teacher, and other team members to identify the student's swallowing and feeding skills
- Functioning as the swallowing and feeding case manager for students on their caseload with behavioral feeding disorders with sensory concerns
- Attending IEP meetings as a member of the IEP committee for students with swallowing and feeding disorders
- Giving input on feeding, sensory issues, positioning and adaptive equipment for the swallowing and feeding plan
- Overseeing the feeding of students including self-feeding, and oral motor skills
- Training the classroom teacher and classroom staff on implementation of the swallowing and feeding plan
- Providing sensory and oral motor therapy when indicated
- Collaborating and consulting with other team members including the teachers, classroom staff, and parents
- Attending ongoing professional development on swallowing and feeding disorders in the school-aged children

Typical Team Role: School Nurse

The school nurse is usually the only "medical" staff on a public school campus and one of the core team members. The nurses bring knowledge of management of a student's health. Nurses are responsible for Individualized Health Plans (IHP), which are a part of the IEP. It is important that they are actively involved in the identification and management of children with swallowing and feeding disorders. The school nurse may be responsible for:

- Monitoring the health of students who are followed by the team
- Writing Individualized Health Plans (IHP) for students followed by the team and training classroom personnel on the IHP

- Training classroom staff on how to react to a choking emergency including individual training on the Heimlich maneuver for each student
- Monitoring a student's weight (when the need is indicated)
- Monitoring a student's lungs periodically during meals when there is a concern of aspiration
- Assisting in contacting physicians in regards to prescriptions, referral, medications, and other medical concerns
- Consulting with parents/guardians, teachers, and therapists regarding health issues
- Helping to secure a detailed, accurate medical history
- Attending IEP meetings as a member of the IEP committee for students with swallowing and feeding disorders
- Attending ongoing professional development on swallowing and feeding disorders in school-aged children

Typical Team Member Role and Responsibility: Special Education Classroom Teacher

Once a swallowing and feeding plan is established, it is then the responsibility of the classroom teacher and her staff to implement the plan. The classroom teacher will have the most contact with the student, will see the student eat the most, and will carry the bulk of the responsibility. It is essential that the core team members provide quality initial and ongoing training for the teacher and the classroom assistants on the swallowing and feeding plan, the IHP, the signs and symptoms of a swallowing and feeding disorder and signs of aspiration, undernutrition, and distress (Homer, 2003). The role of the classroom teacher on the swallowing and feeding team includes the following:

- Overseeing the feeding of the students and implementation of the swallowing and feeding plans on the class roster
- Ensuring that the paraprofessional/classroom assistant prepares the student's cafeteria tray according to the swallowing and feeding plan, including texture modification, liquid management, and food choices, when indicated

- Ensuring that the paraprofessionals/classroom assistants follow each student's swallowing and feeding plan with fidelity
- Recognizing changes in the student's swallowing or feeding and reporting those changes to the case manager
- Following the IHP in the event of a choking incident
- Serving as an information source to other team members on a student's mealtimes, eating habits, and so on
- Keeping the IHP and the swallowing and feeding plan in a location in the classroom that is easily assessable
- Setting up and conducting the IEP as the teacher with IEP authority on the team
- Contacting the swallowing and feeding team case manager when there is a concern or a change in the student's swallowing and feeding
- Following through on recommendations for oral motor stimulation from the SLP and/or OT

Typical Team Member Role and Responsibility: Physical Therapist

Often in the school setting the physical therapist functions as a consultant, training teachers and classroom staff. Children with swallowing and feeding concerns may need the expertise of a physical therapist for the following:

- Addressing postural and mobility issues when they pertain to swallowing and feeding
- Consulting in regards to positioning and adaptive equipment needs related to positioning during mealtimes
- Attending IEP conference when indicated
- Consulting with others on issues pertaining to the student's gross motor skills in relation to swallowing and feeding

Typical Team Member Role and Responsibility: School Administrator

The school administrator, or principal, needs to have an understanding of the issues surrounding children with swallowing and

---

Student Profile: School Administrator Role

School administrators may have a positive or negative effect on the management of students in their schools in small ways that are hard to predict. In this case, there was a classroom of severe profound students that had 5 students all with dysphagia. There were multiple health and safety issues, including a child who sought to put things in his mouth all day long. The teacher did not take seriously the concerns by the swallowing and feeding team and found it challenging to get the paraprofessionals in her classroom to follow the swallowing and feeding plan precautions. The number of students in the class with serious safety issues and concerns, and the ineffective teacher, required the case manager to work intensively with the classroom staff on training. In addition, one of the parents was uncomfortable with the classroom situation and was requesting a 1:1 aide for her child.

The principal at the school was asked by the Special Education Department to choose a teacher to send to a 3 day, non-mandatory workshop on procedural training (unrelated to swallowing and feeding or to students with safety and health issues). The principal chose the teacher in the severe profound class, which would have put a substitute teacher, with minimal training in the safety issues of the students, in the class for 3 days!

Although the school team had kept the principal informed of the concerns, this principal didn't understand the serious issues in the classroom and the importance of the teacher as the person overseeing the class and the staff and, as a result, potentially put the students as risk. The swallowing and feeding team administrator intervened and the principal was instructed by the Special Education Supervisor to choose a different teacher to attend the workshop. This principal did not understand the importance of the trained classroom staff and the seriousness of the situation.

---

feeding disorders. The principal should be aware of the services being provided on the school campus. The school administrator is responsible for:

- Supporting the professionals working with the students with swallowing and feeding disorders
- Serving as a mediator, when indicated, on issues that develop concerning a student's swallowing and feeding
- Attending the IEP conference as the Official Designee Representative (ODR) of the school system

Typical Team Member Role and Responsibility: Cafeteria Manager

The school cafeteria manager will be involved when students with swallowing and feeding disorders need modified or adapted diets in the cafeteria. It is important that the food that is presented to the student complies with the modifications indicated on the student's swallowing and feeding plan. The cafeteria manager is responsible for:

- Ensuring that the food presented on the student's tray follows the recommendations of the swallowing and feeding plan
- Providing a space in the cafeteria kitchen for a station to be set up for altering the texture of foods (e.g., pureeing, etc.) according to the student's plan
- Ensuring that the equipment used to alter the texture of the student's food (e.g., bullet blender) is adequately cleaned

Typical Team Member Role and Responsibility: Paraprofessional/Classroom Assistant

The paraprofessional/classroom assistant operates under the guidance of the special education classroom teacher. The paraprofessional may be asked by the teacher to be responsible for:

- Feeding the student(s) according to the swallowing and feeding plan
- Recording the amount of food eaten and recording behaviors observed
- Preparing/modifying the food presented on the cafeteria tray in the cafeteria station according to the plan

Typical Team Member Role and Responsibility: Medical Team Members

In addition to the school-based team members, the medical team plays a role in the identification and treatment of swallowing and feeding in the school setting. The hospital-based SLP is responsible for conducting the MBSS/VFSS, along with the Radiologist, to help to determine the extent of the swallowing disorder. The hospital SLP will need to work closely with the school-based staff as well as the parents/guardians. The hospital or clinic SLP along with the otolaryngologist is responsible for the FEES test, which also may be used to diagnose the extent of the swallowing disorder. The school staff may need to collaborate and correspond with the student's physicians regarding the student's medical tests, health status, and medical treatment. This may include pediatricians, neurologists, gastroenterologists, pulmonologists, otolaryngologist, and radiologists.

When there are concerns about the student's nutritional status, the district team members may need to consult with a dietician. In districts where a dietician is not employed, this will require working closely with the family as well as getting district approval for a consultation.

Refer to Table 3–1 for a summary of the roles and responsibilities of the team members.

Essential Component: A Working Procedure for Addressing Swallowing and Feeding in the School Setting

"Follow the Forms": Components of a Swallowing and Feeding Team Procedure

The importance of having a system-wide procedure has been stressed. Once a system has a procedure in place, it is essential that the procedure be followed with fidelity. According to St. Tammany Parish School Board Attorney, Robert L. Hammonds, in an opinion dated 1995, "the keys to minimizing liability exposure are planning, procedures, training, and the proper execution of those procedures." The Follow the Forms procedure allows for

Table 3–1. Roles and Responsibilities of School-Based Swallowing and Feeding Team Members

Speech-Language Pathologist	Classroom Teacher
Referral source Serves as case manager Initial identification of students at risk Coordinates assessment/treatment Attends MBSS/VFSS and FEES Writes Swallowing and Feeding Plan Trains teachers and classroom staff Treats oral/pharyngeal phase dysphagia Consults, refers, and monitors esophageal phase dysphagia Monitors feeding and implementation of the Swallowing and Feeding Plan Responds to issues and concerns regarding the student's swallowing disorder	Oversees the feeding of the students on the roster Ensures that the student's cafeteria tray is prepared according to the plan. Ensures that each student's swallowing and feeding plan is implemented with fidelity Follows the IHP in the event of a choking incident Serves as an information source on a student's mealtimes, eating habits, and so on Keeps the IHP and the swallowing and feeding plan in an easily assessable location Sets up and conducts the IEP Recognizes changes and contacts the swallowing and feeding team case manager when there is a concern Follows through on recommendations for oral motor stimulation
Occupational Therapist	**School Nurse**
Referral source Conducts the interdisciplinary observation with the SLP Serves as case manager Oversees the feeding of students Brings knowledge of positioning, sensory awareness and adaptive equipment Trains classroom staff Provides sensory and oral motor therapy Collaborates with other team members Attends the IEP when possible or indicated	Monitors the health of the students Writes the individualized health plan and trains personnel Monitors student's weight Monitors lungs periodically during meals Assists in contacting physicians Consults with parents and teachers Helps to secure the medical history Attends the IEP Monitors nutrition status

continues

Table 3–1. *continued*

Parent/Guardian	Physical Therapist
Shares knowledge of child's feeding habits, food preferences and mealtime environment Provides medical information and history Shares cultural view regarding food and eating Reports changes in child's swallowing and feeding skill or medical status Implements swallowing and feeding goals	Addresses postural skills and mobility issues Addresses positioning and adaptive equipment needs related to positioning for mealtimes. Consults with other team members on issues pertaining to gross motor skills pertaining to swallowing and feeding. Attends the IEP when possible or indicated.
Cafeteria Manager	**Classroom Paraprofessional**
Responsible for providing recommended diet Ensures that the food presented on the student's lunch tray follows the guidelines of swallowing and feeding plan. Allows for a station to be set up for altering the texture of foods (pureeing, etc.) Ensures that the equipment used to alter the texture of the student's food is adequately cleaned	Feeds students according to their plan Records amount of food eaten and behaviors observed during mealtime Prepares and modifies foods for student
School Administrator	**Medical Based Team Members: Physicians, Hospital SLP, Dietician**
Supports the professionals working with the students Serves as mediator Attends IEP meeting as the Official Designee Representative (ODR) of school system	Consults with school case manager on instrumental referrals Conducts instrumental evaluations and writes reports Consults with team regarding referrals, medical and health status, and treatment Consults on nutrition status and recommendations

team members to document the process by using corresponding forms as they identify and address swallowing and feeding concerns throughout the procedure using a step-by-step procedure. Most steps in the procedure have corresponding forms. In addition, the entire procedure is summarized for quick reference on a flowchart (Box 3–1). Each step will be explained in the order that it occurs. This procedure has been used successfully in St. Tammany Parish Schools for 20 years and has been adapted in many school districts throughout the United States.

Identification of Swallowing and Feeding

The initial identification of swallowing and feeding disorders in the schools is made up of three steps: referral, parental input, and interdisciplinary observation. Each step is necessary to accurately identify if a student's swallowing and feeding concerns require the services of the team, to determine where the child is functioning, and if therapeutic intervention is indicated. At the completion of these three steps, the school-based team will have determined what needs to be done to ensure the child's safety during mealtimes at school and if therapy to address oral motor, sensory issues, and other direct intervention is indicated. This initial assessment process is necessary for all students who are suspected of having swallowing and feeding issues; however, the assessment process does not end with this portion of the procedure. Students with swallowing and feeding disorders will need ongoing assessment of their skills.

Step 1: Student Referral to the Team. The first step of any procedure is a process for referring students who exhibit the signs and symptoms of a swallowing and feeding disorder. The Swallowing and Feeding Team Referral Form (see Appendix A) lists signs and symptoms of a student who is at risk for a swallowing and/or feeding disorder. This form should be completed on all students suspected of having a swallowing or feeding disorder. Initially, when a district is beginning their process of identifying students, most referrals will come from school staff such as SLPs, OT, nurses, or classroom teachers. As the school system uses the procedure, this will shift to "child find" students, students new to the district or parent/guardian referral. When a student is

Box 3-1. Swallowing and Feeding
Team Procedure Flowchart

Step 1: Referral
Parent, teacher, SLP, OT, or other refer student to the swallowing and feeding team

Step 2: Parent Input
Contact parent/caregiver and conduct parent interview

Step 3: Interdisciplinary Observations
SLP, OT, nurse, and parent (if possible) conduct interdisciplinary observation at school with teacher

Step 3A: Preconference Following Interdisciplinary Observation	**Step 3B: Preconference Following Interdisciplinary Observation**
Dysphagia/Safety Concerns	Behavioral Feeding Concerns
Preconference may include SLP, OT, nurse, classroom teacher, and parent/guardian	Referral to behavior team
Team members review and discuss parent interview and observations and follow up on medical concerns.	Preconference includes behavior team member, SLP, and OT
Write interim swallowing/feeding plan	Conduct behavior team consent and observation
Write interim emergency plan	
Train classroom staff on both plans	
Initiate swallowing/feeding plan and emergency plan	

Step 4: IEP Conference

IEP Conference set up by teacher with IEP authority and meeting held

Attended by: parent, teacher, SLP, OT, nurse, and administrator

Discuss: swallowing and feeding concerns, additional testing indicated, diet modifications, release of information, referral.

Step 5: Instrumental Examination Referral

MBSS/VFSS/FEES set up and conducted if indicated. Physician referral for additional medical information secured.

Step 6: Review, Revision, and Retraining of the Swallowing/Feeding and Emergency Plans

Review and revise swallowing and feeding plan and emergency plan

Retrain classroom staff

Step 7: Cafeteria Management and Meal Modifications at School

Request prescription for school meal modification from parents/physician

Meet with cafeteria manager to alter school diet

Step 8: Interventions and Treatment

Initiate swallowing and feeding plan

Monitor swallowing and feeding and initiate therapeutic intervention going through the initial evaluation process for special education services, the evaluation team will need to consider the student's swallowing and feeding skills as part of that evaluation. Most states have a Child Find initiative for children approaching 3 years old to 5 years old. Many new referrals will be identified at the time of this initial evaluation. The evaluators should have the training and experience to identify a swallowing and feeding disorder. In all types of referrals, whether a new student, parent request, or school staff concern, the first step is to complete the referral form and to send it to the swallowing and feeding team administrator to begin the process. A copy of the referral should be kept in the student's special education folder.

Step 2: Parental/Guardian Interview. Feeding a child is one of the most important responsibilities of a parent/guardian. There are many emotions involved when a child has difficulty eating. It is extremely important that the school-based team involve the parents/guardians in the process from the very beginning. The Parental/Guardian Interview Form (see Appendix D) is used to gather historical information about a child's feeding and food preferences. Ideally an interview would be done in person; however, in some cases it may be necessary to conduct the interview over the phone. As a last resort it can be sent home for the family to complete. You will get more accurate information when you have the parent sitting in front of you and can read their body language in conjunction with their words. Because the form is extremely detailed, it may be beneficial to send home the blank form for the parent/guardian to review and begin to complete prior to the interview meeting.

One of the most important components of a swallowing and feeding team is a system for open and active communication with the parent/guardian. Parents/guardians provide invaluable knowledge about their children regarding feeding habits at home, medical history, cultural considerations, and personality characteristics. They are the experts on their children and, in many instances, have figured out the safest way to feed them. By respecting parents'/guardians' knowledge, you establish their role on the problem-solving team and often avoid contentious situations. There will always be cases where parent/guardians are uncooperative or make requests that do not seem to be in the student's best interest; however, in the majority of cases parents/guardians are caring and loving and want the best for their children (Homer, 2004).

The parents/guardians play a key role in evaluating the student's swallowing and feeding skills by providing the school team with information on how the child eats at home and informing the team on the students feeding history. They also play an important role in carrying over the feeding skills that their child learns at school. This first contact with the parents/guardians regarding feeding will set the stage for a strong collaborative relationship with the family. For more information on working with parents/guardians and families see Chapter 8.

Step 3: Interdisciplinary Observation of Swallowing and Feeding. Once it has been established that there are swallowing and feeding concerns through the referral and parent/guardian interview, an in-depth observation and assessment of the student eating at school will be necessary to determine the extent of the issues and concerns as well as to determine what strategies may be effective. An examination of the student's oral structures and function should be done prior to the observation. Step 3 has some subcomponents that branch off depending on the findings. It begins with the interdisciplinary observation, which is equivalent to the clinical evaluation of swallowing used in other settings (ASHA, 2000). This observation provides information on how to feed the child safely including positioning, diet and food preparation, equipment, and special precautions. The observation may occur in multiple settings such as the cafeteria and the classroom. The team will choose a time when the members are able to watch the child during lunch. The classroom staff will initially feed the student in the same way as he or she is fed normally. The swallowing and feeding team members will then direct the feeding to determine if there are strategies that will help to make the student's mealtime safer and more efficient. The team will try different strategies and modifications to determine how to safely feed the student at school. The Interdisciplinary Observation Form (see Appendix E) may be used to document the observations and to guide the evaluation. One member of the team, in most cases the case manager, will document on the form what is observed. The form includes the observation of liquids presented, foods presented, behavioral observations, and sensory observations. The team will try different strategies to determine how to feed the child safely. This may include altering textures, liquids, size of bolus, and location of presentation. The interdisciplinary observation determines the following:

- Does the student have a swallowing and feeding concern that warrants being followed by the swallowing and feeding team?
- If the student needs to be followed by the team, what specifically are the concerns and what strategies for feeding will be most effective to establish a safe swallowing and feeding plan for the student?
- If there are medical concerns, does the nurse need to follow up on those issues? Will the team need to follow up with a physician to rule out issues such as gastro esophageal reflux disorder, medication issues, and so forth?
- Does the child present with a behavioral component that needs to be addressed? Is that the only feeding concern, or are there physical and/or sensorimotor concerns in addition to the observed behavioral issues?

Once the team observation is completed, the team will use the information gathered for a pre-IEP conference to determine swallowing and feeding recommendations.

Step 3A: Pre-IEP Conference When There Are Dysphagia/Safety Concerns. A Pre-IEP Conference is part of Step 3, but is divided into two sections. Step 3A immediately follows the interdisciplinary observation and occurs when the student has dysphagia and safety concerns following the referral, parent interview, and interdisciplinary observation. This conference is documented on the Pre-IEP Conference Form (see Appendix F). The team members who conducted the observation will meet to discuss what the concerns are and to draft an interim Swallowing and Feeding Plan Form (see Appendix B). Note that this form will be used again in Step 6. Once it has been determined that a student needs intervention to ensure that he or she is fed safely at school, then the team must put a safe feeding plan in place. Once the plan has been written, the SLP and/or the OT will work with the classroom staff to train them on how to implement the plan. This step is important because the professionals who have training in swallowing and feeding disorders will not be feeding the student on a daily basis. It is essential that classroom staff members responsible for feeding the student know how to follow the plan. Once the staff has been adequately trained, the training is documented on the swallowing and feeding plan form with a signature and date verifying that the training was completed. This documentation helps to ensure that every classroom staff member has been sufficiently trained to safely feed the student. It is the teacher's responsibility to make sure that the swallowing and feeding plan is followed with fidelity and attention to detail. The case manager makes sure that the teacher and her staff knows and understands the plan and is able to implement it. The swallowing and feeding plan should be kept in a confidential place with easy access for quick reference.

The school nurse, following the preconference, writes an individualized health plan (IHP) or emergency plan. This plan describes the medical issues that the classroom staff needs to be aware of and a plan of action should an emergency occur. The nurse will train the classroom staff on the implementation of the IHP. This form is part of the IEP form and will vary state to state. An example is if a child has weak oral motor skills and needs a choking plan. The nurse would train the staff to do the Heimlich maneuver on the student in the case of an emergency. The steps leading up to the need for the Heimlich maneuver would also be in the health plan. This plan will ultimately become part of the student's IEP and should also be kept in a place in the classroom that is easily accessible to the classroom staff. The classroom teacher is responsible for implementation of the plan when there is an emergency. The school nurse and the swallowing and feeding case manager should be contacted whenever there is an emergency situation that is related to a student's swallowing and feeding.

Step 3B: Pre-IEP Conference and Observation to Address Behavioral Feeding Concerns. When a child exhibits behavioral and/or sensory motor feeding issues then a Pre-IEP Conference that specifically addresses the behavior concerns is indicated. When it is evident following the referral, parent interview, and the interdisciplinary observation that the student clearly has a behavioral component to his feeding, then it will be necessary to arrange a pre-IEP conference that may include members of the district's behavioral intervention team. Many school districts will have a team that addresses the unique behavioral issues that surround some students with autism, Down syndrome, and other disorders. The behavior team needs to attend the preconference for these students so the meeting may need to take place at a later date rather than immediately following the Interdisciplinary Observation. If the student has a dysphagia-based swallowing and feeding disorder in addition to the behavioral component, then Step 3A will be completed and 3B will occur when the behavior committee member can attend the conference to address the behavioral issues. Many times there are a number of different issues occurring and not one issue in isolation. It is important that all of the student's swallowing, feeding, and health issues be addressed following the interdisciplinary observation. The swallowing and feeding team will want to continue to work closely with the family as they go through this process. When there is a behavioral component there are often emotional issues that may need to be considered.

When addressing students who have behavioral feeding issues, the district team will need to rule out medical issues and complications that may be present. This will require close communication with the family. Once this preconference is completed, then the team will need to set up a behavioral observation.

Continuation of Step 3B: Observation of the Student With Behavioral Feeding Concerns. Children who exhibit symptoms of behavioral feeding disorders may need an extra step. It is important that the student's feeding developmental skills be assessed, including sensory development, oral motor skill development, medical history and conditions, as well as the swallowing anatomy and physiology. There needs to be a determination of all of these issues to be able to design an effective treatment strategy. Students, who have behavioral feeding disorders with the absence of dysphagia, will require the involvement of a behavioral specialist or Board Certified Behavior Analyst (BCBA). An observation of the student with behavioral concerns should occur not only during mealtimes or snacks, but also in his or her classroom to determine the extent of the behaviors. The behavioral specialists in the schools will be able to determine if the behaviors are consistent with other behaviors in the classroom or if they are unique to feeding. The behavior specialist will also design a plan for extinguishing the behaviors based on the ongoing information collected. A behavior plan that addresses the feeding will be written and the classroom staff trained by the behavioral specialists. In cases where the student has sensory and/or motor issues in addition to the behaviors, the SLP and OT will write a swallowing and feeding plan that addresses those issues as well as the behavior concerns. Chapter 6 discusses management issues with this population. The behavior observation may occur before or after the IEP conference depending on the availability of the behavior specialist, but for these purposes is listed on the flowchart as 3B.

Implementation of Swallowing and Feeding Services

Once it has been determined that the student needs to be followed by the swallowing and feeding team then the implementation phase of the procedure begins. The implementation phase, while primarily addressing how the student will be fed safely and efficiently at school, may also include additional assessment when indicated. The steps in the implementation phase include the following: IEP conference, food and meal preparation, training classroom staff, monitoring and therapeutic intervention, and ongoing assessment and plan revision. In addition, when indicated, medical referrals, observation of behavior feeding, and revision of the swallowing and feeding and individualized health plan.

Step 4: IEP Conference. The IEP conference in school systems serves to identify the needs of students and to design a plan for addressing their needs within the academic context. Once it has been determined that the student needs to be followed by the swallowing and feeding team, then an IEP conference must be held to add the information and to determine the plan. The special education teacher in most cases will be the teacher with IEP authority and will be responsible for setting up the meeting. The meeting should include the following members: the parent, special education teacher, regular education teacher, administrator, SLP, OT, school nurse, and behavior specialist (if indicated). The meeting is held to accomplish the following:

- Discuss the findings of the referral, parent/guardian interview, and interdisciplinary observation
- Review the established plan for feeding the student at school and make revisions if indicated
- Review the established individualized health plan and have parent sign the plan
- Discuss and have parents sign the release of information forms that allow the district to give and receive information from the student's physicians
- Discuss and determine if an instrumental evaluation is indicated (MBSS/VFSS/FEES), and, if so, get information on getting a prescription from the physician for the referral
- Request that the parents/guardians get the Prescription of School Meal Modification Form (see Appendix G) signed by the student's physician

The General Student Information section of the IEP should describe the student's swallowing and feeding concerns and indicate how the district will implement the plan. In many cases when a student moves from one school district to another only official documents, such as the student's special education evaluation and IEP, will be sent to the receiving district; therefore, a brief summary of the swallowing and feeding plan should be included in the Health Needs section of the GSI. In some cases, the students will need speech-language therapy and/or occupational therapy to address oral motor and/or feeding issues. Oral motor and/or feeding goals would be added to the instructional page and the program services pages of the IEP. The IEP is an essential step in documenting the swallowing and feeding team plan for feeding the student at school. It is also an opportunity to engage the parents in the plan and its implementation.

Step 5: Instrumental Examination Referral and Physician Referral. Following the IEP, if the committee decides that the student needs further medical follow-up, it will be necessary to secure referrals for an instrumental examination, a meal modification prescription, and/or physician consultation. The school team will need to work with the parents/guardians to obtain these referrals.

Many students in the school system have oral phase dysphagia and a safe swallowing and feeding plan can be written based on the evaluations done at the school and the information gathered from the parents/guardians. In some cases, however, the district will need additional information to accurately assess the safety of a student's swallowing. There may be cases where a student's safety and the efficiency of the swallow during meals remains a question. This could be due to aspiration; a change in the student's signs and symptoms, which may be inconsistent with the Interdisciplinary Observation done previously, or the student may be at risk for failure to thrive (ASHA, 2004). Students who come to a district with a history of dysphagia may also be considered candidates for an instrumental examination. Recommendations for a MBSS/VFSS or FEES examination present a challenge for the school district team. The team will need to work closely with parents/guardians to secure a physician prescription for the study. Having a positive working relationship with the parents/guardians makes this process go more smoothly. If a student needs to be referred for an MBSS/VFSS or FEES, it is more efficient for the school system to set up the study directly with the hospital. This allows the school system to arrange and facilitate payment of the portion of the study not covered by private insurance or Medicaid. It also allows the district to arrange the study at a time that would include the district's swallowing and feeding team representative (typically the case manager) to attend the study. The school-based SLP can work with the hospital SLP to ensure that the district's questions and concerns are all answered.

Prior to the study, the district case manager contacts the hospital SLP to discuss the student and the school district's concern. This can only be done once the release of information form has been signed and the orders received. The communication between the medically based team and the school-based team is essential to ensure interactive decision making in the area of dysphagia (Arvedson, 2001). It is the responsibility of the school district swallowing and feeding team case manager to make sure that there is communication with the medical team when it is indicated. In addition to calling the hospital SLP, the case manager will complete and send to the hospital SLP, a Pre-Instrumental Examination Information Form (see Appendix H). This form provides the hospital team with the information they will need to be able to answer the questions presented by the school-based team. The information on the form informs the hospital SLP of the clinical observations that had been recorded during the initial determination of a swallowing and feeding concern. It also provides information on how the student is currently being fed at school and lists the information that the school team would like to get from the study. Talking to the hospital SLP and providing the pre-instrumental examination information prior to the study can make the difference between a successful study and a study that does not provide the information the district needs. The school district's case manager attends the study to ensure that the study addresses the school system's issues and concerns as well as providing support for the parents/guardians, the student, and the hospital SLP (Homer, 2008).

Most instrumental examination referrals will be for the MBSS/VFSS examination, but in some cases a FEES test will be the choice to acquire the information needed. Some students will not be able to tolerate or participate in an MBSS/VFSS examination. The FEES may be chosen when a student is unable to tolerate barium, is too medically fragile for a MBSS/VFSS, or is fed in a manner that obstructs the view for an MBSS/VFSS. The endoscopic assessment provides the following information:

- Identification of normal and abnormal anatomy and physiology of the swallow as can be viewed with the endoscope
- Evaluation of the integrity of airway protection during swallowing
- Evaluation of the effectiveness of postures, maneuvers, bolus modifications, and so forth in improving swallowing safety and efficiency
- Recommendations regarding the optimum delivery and maintenance of nutrition and hydration (ASHA, 2004)

Collaboration of the parents/guardians, the school system swallowing and feeding team case manager, and the hospital team will provide optimum information and results for the student. Once the instrumental examination is completed, the school system team will discuss the results and revise the swallowing and feeding plan, if a change is needed. The team's focus is to establish a safe and efficient feeding plan for the student at school. It is always beneficial if the parents/guardians follow the same plan at home; however, the school team is required to follow the safe feeding plan established, regardless of whether or not the family is following the school plan. When a parent requests that the team feed the child in a manner that the team has determined is not safe, the school-based team has the responsibility to do what is in the best interest of the child at school.

Physician Referral. In some cases it will be necessary to communicate directly with the student's physician. Contact the parents/guardian to discuss the need for a conversation with the child's physician. A release of information form must be signed by the parent/guardian prior to contacting the physician's office. Always document any conversations with the parents/guardians and physician's or their office staff.

Step 6: Review, Revision, and Retraining of the Swallowing and Feeding Plan and/or Individualized Health Plan. Following the IEP conference, the medical referral and/or the behavioral observation, it may be necessary to revise the swallowing and feeding plan and/or the Individualized Health Plan depending on the information gathered. If revisions are necessary then the classroom staff needs to be retrained on the changes. The swallowing and feeding case manager is responsible for the revision and retraining of the swallowing and feeding plan and the school nurse assigned to that student is responsible for the IHP and the retraining.

Step 7: Cafeteria Management and Meal Preparation at School. Once the IEP conference has been completed and a swallowing and feeding plan has been written, the swallowing and feeding case manager will need to work to ensure that the child receives the food that he or she is able to eat according to the plan. There are two, equally important things that must be done at this point:

1. The case manager will meet with the cafeteria manager to determine which foods are appropriate for that

student. It is common for school meal plans to have a monthly menu of meals that repeats every month. This menu should be reviewed and adjusted by the cafeteria manager and the swallowing and feeding case manager. It will be necessary to go through each day and cross out foods that the student cannot have (e.g., pizza for a child on a puree diet) and then a substitute of equal nutritional value is determined. (e.g., on Wednesday they have pizza, but on Tuesday they had chicken nuggets. The chicken nuggets can be pureed so the cafeteria staff will save the nuggets for the student for Wednesday.) This process is repeated for each day and the cafeteria manager is then responsible for making sure that the food presented on the student's tray in the cafeteria is nutritious and follows the swallowing and feeding plan. The cafeteria manager will also assist in setting up a blending station for the classroom staff to prepare the food that is presented on the student's tray according to the child's swallowing and feeding plan. The cafeteria staff is responsible for washing and sterilizing the equipment used to blend the food. See Chapter 7 for additional information on child nutrition at school.

2. The cafeteria program in the schools requires a physician's prescription for school meal modification. This is a procedure in school districts, which is followed whenever a child needs a special diet such as for diabetic children, and children with food allergies. It is recommended that if the child's swallowing and feeding plan has a meal alteration that requires the food be changed before it is put on the student's cafeteria tray, then it is necessary to get a prescription from the physician. If the food is altered after it is on the tray, then a script is not needed. (e.g., puree is done in the cafeteria before the food is put on the child's tray; chopped is done after the food is put on the tray and does not need a script.)

Immediately following the IEP conference, the swallowing and feeding case manager will begin the process of getting a Prescription of School Meal Modification Form (see Appendix G) signed by the student's physician; however, the recommendations are implemented immediately to ensure the safety of the student during mealtimes at school . The school nurse and parents/guardians may assist with this process. The case manager should include the findings of the interdisciplinary observation so that the physician is aware of the student's issues and of the recommended diet. The meal modification script needs to be done yearly, or when there is a major change.

Step 8: Intervention and Treatment. At this point in the procedure, the student has a safe swallowing and feeding plan, the classroom staff has been trained in both the swallowing and feeding plan and the Individualized Health Plan and the cafeteria is prepared to provide the student's meals according to the swallowing and feeding plan. This step in the procedure now depends on the needs of each individual student. The professionals on the team will be responsible for setting up an intervention and/or treatment plan for each student. All students will need to be put on a monitoring schedule where the therapist has a scheduled time dedicated to monitoring the student's swallowing and feeding to ensure that the student is being fed correctly and that the plan is being followed with fidelity and is appropriate. This monitoring process is discussed in detail in Chapter 5. Some students will benefit from direct intervention with goals such as progressing to a more normalized diet, improving the oral preparation phase, improving feeding skills, and/or addressing sensory issues.

Documentation of the Procedure

Providing almost any service in a public school system requires some form of documentation of the service provided. Documentation of the swallowing and feeding procedures are extremely important and is an essential part of the procedure.

Record of Services Provided. A child with a swallowing and/or feeding disorder is often at risk for health and safety issues. Once you have a procedure in place that the entire district will be utilizing, it is essential that you document that the procedure was followed with fidelity. By "Following the Forms" in this procedure you are not only going through the procedure and ensuring that the identification and implementation of treatment of the swallowing and feeding disorder have occurred but you have documentation throughout the process. The forms are designed to offer a guide through the process as well as a means for documenting what the team looked at and considered and how the student performed. This record of the procedure will offer support if the team is ever questioned as to how decisions were reached. The input from the parents and other team members are well documented on the forms as well as the record of classroom staff training, interdisciplinary participation, and consideration of the student's issues and concerns.

Continuation and Management of Services

In addition to recording the process, the forms provide essential information, such as when a student changes districts or schools, that is needed to continue the student's swallowing and feeding program without having to duplicate the services. The Swallowing and Feeding Team Procedure Checklist will help the case manager to keep track of each step of the procedure and will provide a record of when each step was done (see Appendix I).

Swallowing and Feeding Team Student Transfer Procedures

Students who are followed by the swallowing and feeding team will often move from one school to another either during the course of a school year or at the end of the year. Either situation requires that the receiving school and the swallowing and feeding case manager is alerted to the fact that a student with swallowing and feeding concerns is at their school site and that records and information are also transferred. It is recommended that a sticker be added to the outside of a student's folder indicating that the student is followed by the swallowing and feeding team. A sticker on the folder will serve as another way to ensure that the receiving team members are notified. Use the Swallowing and Feeding Team Case Manger Transfer Form (see Appendix C) to notify the SLP or OT who serves as the receiving case manager. This form identifies the student, the current case manager, and current school as well as the receiving case manager and receiving school.

Beginning of The School Year Procedure

At the beginning of each school year, students move to different schools such as from elementary to middle school or they may transfer to a different school site. It is important that the student's swallowing and feeding information is at the student's school for the first day the student attends. It is suggested that at the beginning of the school year the swallowing and feeding team administrator distribute to the SLPs and OTs a roster containing the names of all the students who they will serve as case manager for swallowing and feeding as well as a list of the assigned case managers for each school.

The receiving case manager checks to see if the swallowing and feeding students who were transferred to their school are registered there and are at the school. When receiving a new student, the following procedures should be followed:

1. If the referred student is at school, the case manager immediately refers to the student's swallowing and feeding plan, observes the student, and trains the teachers and paraprofessionals/classroom assistants. It is important that this is done the first day of school.
2. If the student is not at the assigned case manager's school, then the case manager finds out where the student is attending school. Most districts today have a student information system (SIS) that stores information about the students in the district. The SIS may help the case manager locate the school the student is enrolled. The case manager then uses the list of case managers to determine who the manager should be, notify the new manager and transfer the student's records to the school.

Every district has a process for transferring school records, however, the swallowing and feeding information must be transferred as quickly and efficiently as possible to ensure the student's safety at school. The Swallowing and Feeding Team Case

Manger Transfer Form (see Appendix C) is used to notify the receiving case manager.

Student Transfers to a Different School During the School Year

When a student moves from one school to the other during the school year, the entire team, depending on the team model chosen (see Chapter 1) may change and a new swallowing and feeding team case manager may need to be assigned. Use the following procedure to make this transfer:

1. Refer to the Swallowing and Feeding Case Manager listing (see Table 1–3 in Chapter 1) to determine which case manager is assigned to the student's new school.
2. Call the new case manager to inform him or her that they will be receiving a new swallowing and feeding student and to discuss the case with them.
3. Send a copy of the completed Swallowing and Feeding Team Case Manger Transfer Form (see Appendix C) along with a current Swallowing and Feeding Plan Form (see Appendix B) to the new case manager.
4. Send a copy of the Transfer Notice and swallowing and feeding plan to the swallowing and feeding team administrator.

Discharge From the Swallowing and Feeding Team

There are situations when a student may no longer need the services of the swallowing and feeding team. A student should be discharged from the swallowing and feeding team when the following occurs:

- The student is able to eat a variety of foods and textures appropriate for his developmental stage.
- The student is not tube fed.
- The student does not need any special, adaptive equipment for feeding.
- The student is not on a special diet such as puree, mechanical-chopped, and so on

- The student is not a health risk for failure to thrive due to poor nutrition as a result of the inability to swallow or chew, behavior, or other concerns.
- The student does not need special instructions for mealtimes.

To determine if a student is ready to be discharged from the swallowing and feeding team, the case manager should talk to other team members including the classroom teacher, parent/guardian, OT, SLP, and nurse. The decision to discharge a child is always a team decision.

Once the decision has been made by the team to discharge the student, the following process should be followed:

- The case manager should write in the comment section of the IEP, the status of the student including an explanation of why he or she is being discharged from the swallowing and feeding team.
- The parent/guardian must initial the change on the IEP. The parent/guardian has been part of the team process of deciding to discharge the student and should already be aware of the decision.
- A copy of the page of the IEP with the comment stating that the student is being discharged should be sent to the swallowing and feeding administrator and the student will be taken off the list of swallowing and feeding students.

Summary of Swallowing and Feeding Team Procedure

Addressing swallowing and feeding in a school setting is a complex process that is made possible by a district having a swallowing and feeding team procedure. The procedure ensures that students have a plan for safe mealtimes, that district personnel are prepared to address the student's needs, and that they know and understand their roles. Following the procedure provides a process for documenting that the district addressed the safety and feeding issues of each student and provides system support for the employees who are addressing swallowing and feeding. This procedure may be adapted for almost any size district in any state, making adjustments for local regulations.

References

American Speech-Language-Hearing Association. (2000). *Clinical indicators for instrumental assessment of dysphagia* [Guidelines]. Retrieved from http://www.asha.org/policy

American Speech-Language-Hearing Association. (2004). *Role of the speech-language pathologist in the performance and interpretation of endoscopic evaluation of swallowing: guidelines* [Guidelines]. Retrieved from http://www.asha.org/policy

Arvedson, J. (2001). Pediatric clinical feeding and swallowing evaluation. *Swallowing and Swallowing Disorders (Dysphagia), 10*(2), 17–23.

Arvedson, J., & Brodsky, L. (2002). *Pediatric swallowing and feeding: Assessment and management* (Rev. ed., pp. 85–89). San Diego, CA: Singular.

Homer, E. (2003). An interdisciplinary team approach to providing dysphagia treatment in the schools. *Seminars in Speech and Language, 24*(3), 215–227.

Homer, E. (2004). Dysphagia in the schools: One district's proactive approach to providing services to children. *Perspectives on Swallowing and Swallowing Disorders (Dysphagia), 13*(1), 7–9.

Homer, E. (2008). Establishing a public school dysphagia program: A model for administration and service provision. *Language, Speech, and Hearing Services in Schools, 39*, 177–191.

Homer, E., Bickerton, C., Hill, S., Parham, L., & Taylor, D. (2000). Development of an interdisciplinary dysphagia team in the public schools. *Language, Speech, and Hearing Services in Schools, 31*, 62–75

4

Recognizing Swallowing Impairment in the School Setting

Memorie M. Gosa

Key Points

1. Anatomy and physiology of the respiratory system
2. Anatomy and physiology for swallowing
3. Clinical signs and symptoms of aspiration
4. Consequences of aspiration
5. Assessment of swallowing function with diagnostic imaging

Introduction

The school years are a time of amazing growth and development. Appropriate physical growth and neurologic maturation during childhood is dependent on safe and adequate nutritional intake. Children with swallowing and feeding problems often have difficulty managing both the safe and adequate aspects of oral intake. Impaired swallow function can result in aspiration.

Aspiration, entry of food or liquid below the level of the vocal folds, is a known cause of pulmonary morbidity and mortality in children. It is imperative that professionals who provide services to children with swallowing and feeding difficulties be keenly aware of the anatomical and physiological features of respiration and swallowing regardless of their practice setting. When abhorrent swallowing and feeding skills are suspected, referrals and recommendations for further testing may be necessary. This chapter focuses on establishing knowledge of typical respiratory and swallowing function and how to recognize and document deviant functioning to make appropriate referrals for speech-language pathologists managing children with dysphagia in a school setting.

Respiratory Anatomy and Physiology

Anatomy

The respiratory system is traditionally divided into two parts, the upper and lower respiratory tracts. The upper respiratory tract includes the nose, nasal passages, pharynx, and larynx. Oxygen is drawn into the body through the nose and travels through the nasal passages, through the nasopharynx, oropharynx, and into the larynx as it passes through the hypopharynx. It is imperative that the structures of the upper respiratory tract be sufficiently patent to allow for adequate intake of oxygen. The nose and nasal cavities serve to moisten, warm, and filter the air before it enters the lower respiratory tract. The larynx serves as the gateway to the lower respiratory tract. Through its valving action, the larynx can open to allow free passage of air into the trachea or it can close to prevent foreign bodies, including food and liquid, from entering the trachea. Closing the larynx also makes possible thoracic fixation for situations that require increased abdominal pressure, such as defecation or heavy lifting (Ball, Bindler, & Cowen, 2010; Bosma & Showacre, 1975; Marieb, 1995; Zemlin, 1998).

The lower respiratory tract includes the trachea, bronchi, bronchioles, and the lungs. The lungs are inclusive of the respiratory bronchioles, alveolar ducts, alveolar sacs, and alveoli. The lower respiratory tract transitions from being a conduit or tube for oxygen to the lungs where gas exchange takes place. The trachea extends from the larynx in a single column until it divides, usually at the level of the fifth thoracic vertebra in the adult, into the right and left main stem bronchi. The main stem bronchi connect the trachea to the right and left lungs with the right bronchus being slightly larger in diameter. The right bronchus supplies the larger lung and has less of an angle at the carina (rigid structure at the place of division) than the left lung. Therefore, it is more common for foreign bodies to be found in the right main stem bronchi and lung than the left. The bronchi continue to divide to form the bronchial tree. The left bronchus divides into two secondary bronchi and the right bronchus divides into three secondary bronchi. These secondary bronchi supply each of the lobes in the left (two lobes) and right (three lobes) lungs. The secondary bronchi then divide into tertiary bronchi that supply individual lung segments. The tertiary bronchi divide into microscopic segments called bronchioles. The histologically distinguishable bronchioles continue to divide giving rise to the terminal bronchioles. The terminal bronchioles mark the end of the conducting zone and the transition into the respiratory zone. The terminal bronchioles are responsible for the production of surfactant, which is a secretion that decreases surface tension and allows the lungs to expand during inspiration and prevents them from collapsing during expiration (Ball et al., 2010; Marieb, 1995; Zemlin, 1998).

Continuing into the respiratory zone, the next division of the respiratory tree brings about the respiratory bronchioles and they divide into many alveolar ducts. The alveolar ducts then terminate into alveolar sacs and individual alveoli. The alveoli are the functional units of the lungs and it is here that gas exchange takes place. The alveoli can be thought of as small cavities. An intricate network of capillaries surrounds the alveolar membranes and allows an exchange of oxygen from inhalation with carbon dioxide and metabolic waste from the blood. The carbon dioxide is then expelled from the body during exhalation. The alveoli are made from elastic and collagen fibers. The elasticity of the alveoli and the presence of surfactant allows them to expand as they are filled with air during inhalation and then recoil quickly back to their resting position during exhalation (Ball et al., 2010; Marieb, 1995; Zemlin, 1998).

The lungs, heart, and bronchial tree are contained within the thoracic cavity. The ribs, sternum, vertebral column, and diaphragm define the space of the thoracic cavity. The diaphragm separates the thoracic cavity from the abdominal cavity. The lungs are connected to the thorax via the pleural linkage. The visceral pleura membrane covers the lungs and the parietal pleura membrane covers the thorax. Pleural fluid separates these two connected membranes, creating a hydrostatic force that allows them to move easily over each other but makes them very difficult to separate. The linkage of the lungs to the thorax results in the lungs maintaining partial inflation even when at rest and it prevents the thorax from reaching its full volume potential. The pleural linkage balances these two tendencies keeping the lung partially inflated at 40% of the total lung capacity when at rest. This rest state is referred to as the functional residual capacity. It is the connection of the lungs to the ribs that allows for inhalation and exhalation (Ball et al., 2010; Marieb, 1995; Zemlin, 1998).

Physiology

To initiate inhalation, a pressure differential must first exist between the environmental pressure and the alveolar pressure. When the alveolar pressure is below the environmental pressure this creates a pressure gradient allowing air to flow into the lungs. In contrast, when the alveolar pressure is greater than atmospheric pressure a pressure gradient is created that allows for air to flow out of the lungs. Passive and active forces in the body influence alveolar pressure. The elastic recoil forces present in the respiratory system are the passive forces. Active forces are the result of contraction by the respiratory muscles. Inspiration is always the result of muscular action. The diaphragm contracts to increase the volume of the thoracic cavity, thereby reducing the alveolar pressure. The external intercostal muscles contract to lift the ribs up and out and expand the volume of the thoracic cavity. Expiration is primarily a passive force, where the elastic recoil forces of the respiratory system provide sufficient force to move the carbon dioxide out of the lungs. However, expiratory pressure can be added to the passive elastic recoil forces when necessary to expedite exhalation. A number of different muscles that have the collective effect of decreasing the volume of the thorax and compressing the abdomen contribute to active expiratory pressure forces (Ball et al., 2010; Bosma & Showacre, 1975; Marieb, 1995; Zemlin, 1998).

Pediatric Growth and Maturation of the Respiratory System

The components of the respiratory system continue to grow and change until approximately 12 years of age. The diameter of the trachea and other respiratory passages in children is smaller than those of the adult. An adult's tracheal diameter is approximately 20 mm, while a child's airway diameter can be estimated by the size of their pinky finger. This narrowed airway diameter creates greater chance for obstruction from edema that results from infection or other irritants. Additionally, the narrowed conducting zone increases airway resistance causing children to breathe more rapidly to maintain oxygenation when there is additional swelling (Ball et al., 2010; Bosma & Showacre, 1975).

The tracheobronchial tree is complete at birth; however, it continues to grow throughout childhood. At approximately eight years of age, the alveoli begin increasing in both size and quantity until reaching approximately 300 million by 18 to 21 years of age. Additionally, children under six years of age primarily use their diaphragm for inhalation because of the immaturity of the intercostal muscles. Despite the physiologic immaturity of children's respiratory systems, they require greater oxygen consumption than adults due to their higher metabolic rate. Their oxygen consumption increases with respiratory distress and children are more prone to muscle fatigue when utilizing accessory muscles for breathing during respiratory distress (Ball et al., 2010; Bosma & Showacre, 1975).

Anatomy and Physiology of Swallowing

Anatomy

A common pathway for both air and food or liquid is present in human beings and is frequently referred to as the upper aerodigestive tract. The upper aerodigestive tract with its shared pathways for oxygen and nutrition presents many challenges to its structural design. As individual components of the upper aerodigestive tract participate in respiration, phonation, and swallowing they must be able to quickly accommodate for each task's specific needs. For respiration, the upper aerodigestive tract must provide airway patency and lower airway protection against foreign body invasion. In contrast, for swallowing it must provide sufficient propulsive force to move a bolus to the stomach through the esophagus while preventing foreign body ingestion into the larynx and lower airway. Phonation requires continuous modulation of this common pathway to produce various phonemes. To accommodate all of these functions, the upper aerodigestive tract must provide rigidity for respiration, flexibility for pharyngeal constriction to allow for bolus propulsion, and selective modulation (opening and narrowing) of eggressive airflow for phonation. Each task requires a specific advantage that poses a disadvantage for the other tasks that must be accommodated in this space. The upper aerodigestive tract is inclusive of the mouth, pharynx, larynx, and esophagus. Each component serves a specific role in the swallowing process (Brodsky & Arvesdson, 2002; Laitman & Reidenberg, 1993).

The mouth is bounded anteriorly by the lips and inferiorly by the palatoglossal fold (anterior faucial pillar). Its superior borders are the hard and soft palates and its inferior border is the muscular floor of the mouth. The mouth is the intake area for food and liquid and in older infants and adults it can be used for respiration if necessary. It also functions as the main output source for speech with the tongue being the primary articulator for human speech. With downward and forward growth of the mandible and entire facial skeleton, reabsorption of sucking pads, and eruption of primary teeth, there is increased space within the oral cavity, which allows for greater freedom of movement for the tongue. Presence of teeth and increased oral cavity space for greater tongue manipulation leads to an expansion of foods from primarily liquids and puréed to foods that require chewing. Additionally, this growth allows for increased space for resonance and greater freedom of movement for the tongue for more sophisticated articulation. The oral cavity and oropharynx contain a series of lymphatic tissue known as the tonsils. The lingual (on posterior third of tongue), palatal (between faucial pillars), and pharyngeal tonsils/adenoids (posterior pharyngeal wall) together create Waldeyer's ring and provide a circular ring of immunologic protection. The tonsils tend to recede in prominence in adulthood. In infants and children they are more prominent and may become enlarged due to infection (hypertrophy). Tonsillar and adenoid hypertrophy can pose a serious threat to airway patency, promote forward tongue carriage in infants and children, promote open mouth posturing and mouth breathing, create an abnormal swallowing pattern, collect food residuals making feeding uncomfortable and potentially pose a risk for aspiration after the swallow, and create dryness of the lips and oral mucosa. Ankyloglossia (tongue tie) can restrict range of motion for the tongue and can have an undesirable affect on feeding and swallowing competency. Maxilla to mandible relationships must also be considered when considering feeding competency. Malocclusion can create swallowing and articulation problems in addition to cosmetic concerns. Oral habits such as thumb sucking must be considered and ameliorated as necessary in the pediatric population to allow for remediation of malocclusions by orthodontics (Bosma, 1972; Brodsky & Arvesdson, 2002).

The pharyngeal cavity extends from the base of the skull to the inferior border of the cricoid cartilage and is ~12 cm long in the adult. In contrast to the adult, the infant pharyngeal length is considerably shorter. The reduced length of the pharynx in the infant contributes to the reduced hyolaryngeal excursion noted during the infant swallow. Also in the infant, there is a considerably more rounded angle from the mouth to the pharynx. With head and neck growth the angle becomes gradually sharper like that typically associated with an adult. The pharyngeal tube itself is not linear; instead, the pharynx is shaped like a cone with the narrowest tip at the inferior end. In the adult and older child, the pharynx can be divided into three regions.

The nasopharynx is the most superior region and it extends from the cranial base to the hard and soft palate. Its function is purely for respiration and it shares the U-shaped configuration of the other two regions. The entrance to the eustachian tubes is found in the nasopharynx. In the adult, the eustachian tubes are sharply angled to discourage flow of liquid or food into the ear. However, in infants and young children they are not angled and allow for inflow by food or liquid, encouraging ear infection in this population when there is untreated nasopharyngeal back-flow. It is only with head and neck growth seen during the first five years of life that the eustachian tubes achieve their angled positioning. The adenoids are also found in the nasopharynx, and their importance has been previously discussed.

In general, pathology of the nasopharynx can contribute to middle ear infection, decreased nasal resonance, and masking of velopharyngeal dysfunction. The oropharynx extends from the hard and soft palate down to the hyoid bone and includes the base of tongue. This is a shared pathway of nutrition and oxygen. The laryngopharynx represents the most inferior region of the pharynx and it extends from the hyoid bone to the lower border of the cricoid cartilage. It is here in the laryngopharynx that the common pathway ends with food and liquid being shunted into the esophagus and oxygen traveling through the larynx to the lower airway (Bosma, 1972; Brodsky & Arvesdson, 2002; Zemlin, 1998).

The larynx is primarily a respiratory structure. It has evolved to include other functions such as protection to the lower airways during swallowing by preventing food and liquid from entering the trachea, regulating volume and rate of airflow into and out of the lungs for speech production, and the building up of sub glottal pressure for coughing, lifting, defecation, and communication. Table 4–1, Laryngeal Comparisons From Infants to Adults, represents the differences of the infant larynx as compared to the adult larynx. During childhood, growth in the head and neck region transitions the infant laryngeal features into what we commonly observe in the adult larynx (Bosma, Donner, Tanaka, & Robertson, 1986; Crelin, 1973; Newman, 2001; Tutor & Gosa, 2012).

It is because of the differences charted above and the previously described differences in the oral cavity that we see a number of

Table 4–1. Laryngeal Comparisons From Infants to Adults

Laryngeal Differences	Infant	Older Children/Adult
Position	More superior with cricoid cartilage located at C_1–C_3	More inferior with cricoid cartilage located at C_6–C_7 after puberty
Size	1/3 of adult size, and proportionally smaller to the rest of the body as compared to adult	Varies between sexes, usually length between 36–44 mm, transverse diameter between 41–43 mm, antero-posterior diameter between 26–36 mm, and circumference between 112–136 mm
Vocal fold length	4.0–4.4 mm	Varies between sexes usually between 11–21 mm
Vocal folds	Membranous portion makes up less of total length Mucosa is thinner Layered structure is not differentiated Absence of ligamentous structure Absence of collagen in vocal fold muscle Less dense anterior and posterior macula flava fibers—implying less anchoring strength	Clear differentiation between superficial, intermediate, and deep layers of the lamina propria
Thyroid cartilage	Short and broad Closer to the hyoid	Develops laryngeal prominence with thyroid notch (especially in men) at puberty

continues

115

Table 4–1. *continued*

Laryngeal Differences	Infant	Older Children/Adult
Epiglottis	Longer, omega-shaped	Leaf shaped
	May make contact with uvula secondary to superior positioning	
	Softer, less rigid, more easily displaced—as is the entire cartilaginous framework	
Arytenoids	More prominent as compared to adult	Small, triangular shaped cartilages that sit atop the cricoid cartilage
	Aryepiglottic folds are disproportionately large	
Narrowest portion	Cricoid cartilage (subglottic region)	Vocal folds (Glottis)
Reflexes	Foreign body more likely to induce apnea	Foreign body should induce forceful coughing

physiologic differences, particularly in the infant swallow. Those differences are listed below:

- Staging of liquid in the valleculae before the swallow during suckle feeding
- Less hyolaryngeal excursion resulting in small residual seen in valleculae after the swallow
- More frequent swallowing as compared to the adult (Newman, 2001)

The human larynx continues to grow until puberty when it is considered to be fully mature. It is with puberty that the gender differences in the larynx can be seen (Kahane, 1982). The reduced vocal fold length and differences in internal structure coupled with superior pharyngeal positioning also has limiting effects on vocalization range in infants. During physical maturation and development there is a laryngeal and pharyngeal widening that occurs that serves to lengthen the oropharynx and hypopharynx (Bosma et al., 1986; Crelin, 1973; Newman, 2001; Tutor & Gosa, 2012).

The esophagus is also shortened in infants and children as compared to adults. In infants the cricopharyngeal sphincter is known to provide transient relaxation, where in adults it is expected to provide a constant pressure zone to maintain closure. A closed cricopharyngeal sphincter prevents the undesired retrograde movement of food, liquid, and other stomach content into the pharynx, oral cavity, and nasal cavities. Spit-up is fairly common in infants as compared to adults. Spit-up is not of immediate concern; however, frequent vomiting is a concern as this is not a common phenomenon in either infants or adults (Cavataio & Guandalini, 2005). Gastroesophageal reflux disease (GERD) is also a known contributor to undesired feeding and swallowing consequences in childhood. GERD can involve backflow of stomach contents into the esophagus or into the pharynx, both of which can have detrimental effects on feeding and swallowing development.

Throughout childhood, the student is adjusting their feeding performance in response to the physical changes of the upper aerodigestive tract. It is traditionally accepted that by age three, all of the oral motor skills are in place to allow typically developing children to eat like adults. Those skills are refined through practice and exposure to different tastes and textures from a healthy, varied diet. Safe swallowing involves the integration of all the individual features of the upper aerodigestive tract and the respiratory system for adequate oral intake without pulmonary consequences (Morris & Klein, 2000). That process is discussed in the following section.

Physiology

The swallowing process is traditionally divided into three distinct stages: oral stage (with a preparatory and transit phase), pharyngeal stage, and esophageal stage. The oral stage begins as an individual recognizes hunger cues. The hunger cues, triggered by either the smell of food or an empty stomach, activate the salivary glands in preparation for eating. Nutrition, either liquids or foods, enters the body through the oral cavity. A tight lip seal and contraction of the buccal muscles ensure that the food or liquid is held within the oral cavity and that it does not fall into the buccal cavities (space between the cheeks and gums/ teeth). If necessary, the food is masticated and mixed with saliva to form a cohesive bolus for swallowing. Mastication requires mandibular depression and elevation in addition to adequate tongue lateralization. Once adequately prepared for swallowing, the mix of food and saliva is returned to the tongue surface and held there in anticipation of continuing down the upper aerodigestive tract in the next stage of the swallow. If no preparation is necessary, then the bolus is kept on the tongue blade. This first phase of the oral stage of swallowing is voluntary and represents learned behavior in older children and adults. Infants begin to learn this oral preparation phase as they move from sole intake of either breast milk or formula to a diet that includes at first pureed textures then transitioning to solid textured foods over the course of many months. Because it is a voluntary phase, it requires exposure and practice to a variety of food textures to establish the necessary coordination and skills to successfully prepare solid boluses for swallowing (Dodds, 1989; Dodds, Steward, & Logemann, 1990; Ramsey, Watson, Gramiak, & Weinberg, 1955; Tuchman, 1994).

As the bolus sits on the tongue blade, the oral transit phase can be voluntarily initiated. At the initiation of the oral transit phase, there is an initial elevation of the larynx via its connection to the hyoid and an anticipatory shortening of the pharynx that occurs as the tongue tip elevates to begin the anterior to posterior movement of the prepared bolus through the oral cavity toward the pharynx. The tongue blade elevates and pushes against the hard palate in a wave like motion to move the bolus through the oral cavity and into the pharynx. In the mature swallow, as the bolus passes the anterior faucial pillars, the pharyngeal stage of the swallow is initiated (Dodds, 1989; Dodds et al., 1990; Ramsey et al., 1955; Tuchman, 1994).

In the reflexive pharyngeal stage, there is sequential contraction of the pharyngeal constrictors that help to move the bolus inferiorly towards the esophagus. The pharynx is also shortened due to contraction of the longitudinal muscles within the pharynx. The larynx is pulled superiorly and anteriorly under the base of the tongue by the action of the tongue and its connection to the hyoid bone. The larynx also initiates valving at three levels to protect the lower airway from foreign body invasion (Dodds, 1989; Dodds et al., 1990; Ramsey et al., 1955; Tuchman, 1994). The true vocal folds close, followed by the vestibular folds, the arytenoids tilt forward towards the epiglottis, and the epiglottis possibly retro flexes over the laryngeal inlet (Rommel, De Meyer, Feenstra, & Veereman-Wauters, 2003). The elevation of the larynx provides a forward pull on the upper esophagus. The upper esophageal sphincter relaxes and opens. The bolus then enters the esophagus, ending the pharyngeal stage and beginning the esophageal stage (Dodds, 1989; Dodds et al., 1990; Ramsey et al., 1955; Tuchman, 1994).

The closing of the larynx requires a brief pause in the inspiratory or expiratory phase of the respiration cycle. This brief pause is referred to as the swallow apnea. It occurs during the swallowing cycle of all human beings (Kelly, Huckabee, Jones, & Frampton, 2007). The point, at which the respiratory cycle is interrupted, either during inhalation or exhalation, is variable depending on the student's anatomic, physiologic, and neurologic maturation. Additionally, the length of the swallow apnea is variable and is mostly dependent on the volume of bolus being swallowed (Klahn & Perlman, 1999; Preiksaitis, Mayrand, Robins, & Diamant, 1992). The student must have a competent respiratory system to allow for this brief pause in respiration during each swallow, while continuing to meet the oxygen requirements of the body.

During the reflexive esophageal stage, the bolus enters the esophagus via the upper esophageal sphincter and moves through it towards the stomach. The esophagus is a muscular tube that produces a peristaltic wave in response to the bolus. The peristaltic wave pushes the bolus towards the lower esophageal sphincter. The lower esophageal sphincter relaxes and allows the bolus passage into the stomach, ending the esophageal stage of swallowing. The tone of the upper esophageal sphincter varies dependent upon a person's state and head position. Additionally, the upper esophageal sphincter varies its diameter and the time that it remains relaxed depending on the incoming bolus size. Once the bolus passes through the upper esophageal sphincter, it returns to its original tonically closed state and the individual components of the upper aerodigestive tract returns to their rest positions (Dodds, 1989; Dodds et al., 1990; Ramsey et al., 1955; Tuchman, 1994).

This sequence happens continuously during a meal. Each swallow requires the same sequence of events. While the complete sequence of events necessary for normal swallowing are described in sequential summary in this and most texts, many of the events in the normal swallow sequence happen simultaneously or within just milliseconds of each other. A summary of actions, muscles, and cranial nerves involved in the oral and pharyngeal stages is provided in Table 4–2 and Table 4–3.

A full discussion of the neurological control of breathing and swallowing is beyond the scope of this chapter. The author refers the reader to the following reference for further information: Steele, C. M., and Miller, A. J. (2010). Sensory input pathways and mechanisms in swallowing: A review. *Dysphagia*, *25*(4), 323–333.

Signs and Symptoms of Aspiration and Its Respiratory Consequences

Failure of the larynx to keep foreign bodies, such as food and liquid, from entering the lower respiratory tract is referred to as aspiration. Aspiration can occur during reflux events or during swallowing as a component of dysphagia. Lefton-Greif (2008) proposes that the causes of pediatric dysphagia may arise from the following five broad diagnostic categories: (1) neurologic disorders, (2) anatomic abnormalities of the aerodigestive tract, (3) genetic conditions, including syndromes and craniofacial anomalies, (4) conditions affecting suck-swallowing-breathing rhythmicity including congenital malformations of the aerodigestive tract (such as laryngomalacia and choanal atresia), and (5) acquired conditions (such as bronchopulmonary dysplasia

Table 4–2. Oral Stage of Swallowing Summary

	Oral Stage of Swallowing				
	Oral Preparatory Phase			Oral Transit Phase	
Actions	Muscles/Glands	Cranial Nerves	Actions	Muscles	Cranial Nerves
Labial seal	Orbicularis oris buccinator	Facial–VII	Anterior tongue forms a depression to contain the liquid or semi-solid bolus	Intrinsic tongue muscle: Superior longitudinal	Hypoglossal–XII
Movement of bolus around oral cavity for mastication on molar surfaces	Extrinsic tongue muscles: Genioglossus Styloglossus Hyoglossus Palatoglossus	Palatoglossus, Pharyngeal branch of Vagus–X All others, Hypoglossal–XII	Tongue tip elevation to the alveolar ridge	Extrinsic tongue muscle: Styloglossus Intrinsic tongue muscle: Superior longitudinal muscle	Hypoglossal–XII

continues

121

Table 4–2. *continued*

Oral Preparatory Phase			Oral Transit Phase		
Actions	**Muscles/Glands**	**Cranial Nerves**	**Actions**	**Muscles**	**Cranial Nerves**
Mastication	*Mandibular Depression*	Geniohyoid, Hypoglossal–XII	Posterior propulsion of bolus by the tongue	Intrinsic Tongue muscles: Vertical Tranverse Inferior longitudinal Superior longitudinal	Hypoglossal–XII
	Lateral pterygoid	All others, Trigeminal–V			
	Anterior belly of the digastric Geniohyoid				
	Mandibular Elevation				
	Temporalis				
	Masseter				
	Medial Pterygoid				
Mixing with saliva	Sublingual, Submandibular, and Parotid Salivary Glands	Parotid, Glossopharyngeal–IX			
		All others, Facial–VII			

Table 4–3. Pharyngeal Stage of Swallowing Summary

Pharyngeal Stage of Swallowing		
Actions	**Muscles**	**Cranial Nerves**
Soft palate elevation for nasopharyngeal port closure	Levator veli palatini Tensor veli palatini Palatopharyngeus	Pharyngeal branch of Vagus–X
Hyolaryngeal excursion	Mylohyoid Anterior belly of digastric	Trigeminal–V
	Stylohyoid Posterior belly of digastric	Facial–VII
	Palatoglossus	Vagus–X
	Genioglossus Hyoglossus Styloglossus Geniohyoid	Hypoglossal–XII
Laryngeal valving/ closure	Intrinsic laryngeal muscles: Lateral cricoarytenoid Transverse arytenoid Oblique arytenoid Thyroarytenoid Cricothyroid	Vagus–X Superior laryngeal nerve & Recurrent laryngeal nerve Branches
Upper esophageal sphincter relaxation	Cricopharyngeus	Vagus–X
Bolus movement and clearance through the pharynx	Superior pharyngeal constrictor Medial pharyngeal constrictor Inferior pharyngeal constrictor Stylopharyngeus Salpingopharyngeus Palatopharyngeus	Stylopharyngeus, Glossopharyngeal–IX All others, Vagus–X, Pharyngeal branch

and respiratory syncytial virus), and other correlated conditions such as gastroesophageal reflux disease (GERD) and pervasive developmental delay (PDD). Interestingly, four of the above mentioned categories that result in dysphagia in the pediatric population are the direct result of anatomical or physiologic conditions that affect the respiratory system.

Clinical signs and symptoms of aspiration in pediatric populations may include one or more of the following: apnea/bradycardia/acute life threatening events, stridor with feeding, poor weight gain/growth, chronic laryngitis, recurrent episodes of pneumonia, multiple episodes of respiratory infection, and the increased risk of developing chronic lung disease (Tuchman, 1988; Tutor & Gosa, 2012). Children with continuous aspiration may have wheezing that is unresponsive to traditional therapies. Chronic cough is also a common clinical sign of aspiration that can occur during the swallow or from reflux. Aspiration lung disease is a generic term that can refer to any number of clinical syndromes ranging from a single massive aspiration event to chronic lung aspiration. Aspiration lung disease has the potential to cause permanent damage to the developing lungs of children. Pulmonary aspiration (a component of aspiration lung disease) is most commonly the result of dysphagia (swallowing dysfunction), gastroesopheageal reflux disease (GERD), or insufficient management of oral secretions (de Benedictis, Carnielli, & de Benedictis, 2009).

Development of any of the previously mentioned sequelae may result in poor oral intake and subsequent protein energy malnutrition (PEM). PEM frequently results in impairment to the immunologic response of subsequent infections (Tuchman, 1988). In general, dysphagia in the pediatric population has a direct impact on caloric intake and overall nutritional status therefore affecting maturation of all the developing body systems in young children (Newman, 2000). Effective diagnosis and management of dysphagia in the pediatric population is essential to minimizing the detrimental and potentially lethal effects of uncontrolled aspiration (de Benedictis et al., 2009; Newman, 2000). The risk of aspiration during swallowing is the direct result of shared components for deglutition and respiration. When aspiration from dysphagia is suspected, it is essential to refer the student for imaging to provide accurate information about the safety and adequacy of the swallowing response.

Assessment of Swallowing Function
With Diagnostic Imaging

Instrumental assessment is necessary for definitive diagnosis of swallowing dysfunction and aspiration (Lefton-Greif & McGrath-Morrow, 2007). However, instrumental assessment is not necessary in all cases of feeding problems. If a clinician suspects a physiologic problem within the swallow sequence, then an instrumental assessment is necessary to visualize and document the problem within the swallow physiology that is causing the observable symptoms. If a clinician determines that the feeding problem is due to behavioral or sensory aversion, they do not suspect ongoing problems within the swallowing physiology, and there is no concern regarding the safety of the swallow, then an instrumental assessment is not necessary. The clinical assessment and thorough case history are paramount in helping the clinician decide if the student needs to be referred for instrumental assessment. Please review Chapter 3 in this text for a complete description of the clinical assessment and case history interview.

Instrumental assessment requires an order from the physician to the referral site. Communication regarding the family and school swallowing and feeding team's concerns and request for instrumental assessment should be coordinated through the student's dysphagia case manager within the school swallowing and feeding team. Once the instrumental referral assessment appointment has been made, that information should be communicated back to the school. This may require a follow-up phone call or e-mail with the student's family or physician. Instrumental assessment for dysphagia might include the following: modified barium swallow study (MBSS)/Videofluoroscopy (VFSS), fiberoptic endoscopic evaluation of swallowing with or without sensory testing (FEES or FEESST), ultrasonography, manometry, and scintigraphy (Kramer & Eicher, 1993; Lefton-Greif, 2008; Newman, 2000; Tabaee et al., 2006). The most common procedures for evaluation of swallowing function in pediatric populations are the MBSS/VFSS and the FEES(ST). Each test has distinct advantages and disadvantages when considered for students. Both tests not only provide objective information regarding swallowing function and the presence or absence of aspiration, but they also provide information regarding the effectiveness of potential compensatory strategies to assist in accommodating safe swallow.

MBSS/VFSS

The MBSS/VFSS is the only instrumental assessment that provides visualization of the anatomy of the oral cavity, pharynx, larynx, and upper esophagus as well the function and integration of all four areas during the dynamic process of swallowing. This makes it ideal for providing a thorough assessment of swallowing function and of compensatory measures to improve swallowing function (Benson & Lefton-Greif, 1994; de Benedictis et al., 2009; Kramer & Eicher, 1993; Newman, 2000).

Goals of the MBSS/VFSS include objective identification of oropharyngeal swallowing dysfunction, stressing the student's system attempting to recreate the dysphagia symptoms, and evaluating the effectiveness of proposed treatment strategies (Benson & Lefton-Greif, 1994). This is accomplished by age/developmentally appropriate positioning of students within a fluoroscopic suite in a specialized seating device that provides adequate trunk, neck, and head control.

Presentation of test materials and viscosity of test materials are also presented in an age/developmentally appropriate format and should follow a standard protocol (Newman, 2000). The ultimate goal of the MBSS/VFSS is to determine the physiologic cause of the dysphagia symptom (i.e., aspiration, laryngeal penetration, etc.) and then identify the most appropriate treatment strategies to determine the safest and most appropriate intake of calories. Depending on the dysfunction identified in either the oral, pharyngeal, or esophageal phase, compensatory measures may be introduced that are either direct or indirect in nature (Benson & Lefton-Greif, 1994; Newman, 2000). "If the report does not contain the anatomic or physiologic reason for the aspiration or residue (or other symptom) and the interventions attempted to reduce or eliminate these symptoms and their effects, or reasons why they could not be attempted, the study is incomplete" (Logemann, 1998).

FEES/ FEESST

FEES enables direct visualization of soft tissue structures before and after the swallow (de Benedictis et al., 2009). It is a safe assessment for students of all ages including preterm infants (Arvedson, 2008; Leder & Karas, 2000; Willging & Thompson, 2005). The portability of the endoscope and recording equipment make it ideal for assessing students in more natural settings and may be preferred for students that can not easily transfer into the fluoroscopic environment due to limited mobility and dependence on positioning aids (Rees, 2006). The speech-language pathologist or physician passes a small flexible endoscope through the student's nose. The flexible endoscope is positioned for optimal visualization of the hypopharynx and larynx. Test materials are colored to provide improved visualization of the foods and liquids as they are swallowed (Rees, 2006).

During feeding, FEES can identify oropharyngeal dysfunction that occurs before the swallow such as spillover and laryngeal penetration or aspiration. During the swallow, pharyngeal constriction causes white out and briefly disrupts visualization of pharyngeal structures. After the swallow, residual material can be seen and the presence of laryngeal penetration or aspiration from the residue can be noted. Additionally, aspiration during the swallow may be identified with visualization of food or liquid in the trachea after the swallow (Rees, 2006). Treatment strategies can then be tested and a treatment plan made based on information collected from the history, clinical feeding assessment, and FEES.

FEESST gives the examiner information about swallowing dysfunction and then also provides information about the laryngeal adductor reflex (LAR). The LAR is vital for airway protection. The LAR is stimulated by providing controlled air pulses to the aryepiglottic folds through the port of a flexible laryngoscope. The aryepiglottic folds are innervated by the superior laryngeal nerve and by stimulating them with increasing pressure in the form of the air pulse the examiner gains information about the laryngopharyngeal mechanosensitivity. Normal LAR is elicited with less than 4.0 mmHg air pulse pressure; anything greater than that is considered abnormal. Abnormal laryngoharyngeal mechanosensitivity can result from a variety of conditions including gastroesophageal reflux disease and damage to the superior laryngeal nerve (Thompson, 2003; Willging & Thompson, 2005).

The different aspects of the MBSS/VFSS and FEES/FEEST exams are outlined in Table 4–4. The MBSS/VFSS and FEES/FEESST play different and complimentary roles in the evaluation of oropharyngeal dysphagia in pediatric populations (Rees, 2006).

Communication with the medical speech-language pathologist is essential to ensuring that the instrumental exam, either MBSS/VFSS or FEES/FEESST, is beneficial to the student and the school swallowing and feeding team. It is recommended that the school speech-language pathologist communicate with the medical speech-language pathologist before the instrumental exam if possible. However, it may be difficult to identify the medical speech-language pathologist that will actually be performing the instrumental assessment prior to the student's appointment. Appendix J contains a communication tool that can be used to share observations and concerns regarding the student's swallowing issues with the person performing the instrumental assessment. It can be completed by the school swallowing and feeding team with input from the student (if possible) and their family and given to the medical speech-language pathologist by the student's family on the day of the appointment. Ideally, the school swallowing and feeding team will have the chance to either speak to the medical speech-language pathologist or provide him or her with the results of their clinical assessment in writing or by phone prior to the instrumental appointment; however, if that is not possible, using the communication tool in Appendix J will still allow for sharing of concerns and information regarding the student's feeding skills. Sending it with the student on the day of their appointment ensures that it will not get lost or not be received before the instrumental exam.

Financial Considerations of Instrumental Assessment

When referring a student for instrumental assessment, the issue of paying for the procedure must be considered. If a public school student qualifies for special education services under the Individuals with Disabilities Education Act (IDEA), then those

Table 4–4. Differing Aspects of Instrumental Exams for Diagnosing Dysphagia

Exam	What can we see?	What does the student have to eat?	How long will the tests last?	How do I determine which test to request?
VFSS	X-ray images of all four stages of the swallow sequence	Small amounts of barium liquids and powders that may or may not be mixed with real foods	Strict limit of two to four maximum minutes of fluoroscopy time	The two exams are complementary and each offers advantages and disadvantages in the diagnosis of dysphagia. • What are the specific diagnostic questions you would like answered by the exam?
FEES/FEESST	Color images of the soft tissues in the pharynx and larynx before and after the swallow	Real foods of varying consistencies that have food coloring mixed with them (usually blue or green)	No time limit; the scope can remain in place for an entire meal if necessary and tolerated	• What are the student's individual characteristics and which exam do you think they will tolerate best? • What is the availability of each exam in your region? • Consider the student's mobility and positioning needs—there are greater restrictions on the size of wheelchairs and positioning aids allowed during the VFSS

services are to be provided to the student at no cost to the parent. IDEA is not the only source of funding for special education services within the public school system. Turnbull and Turnbull (1997) explain that students must first exhaust all benefits entitled to them from the "payers of first resort" before they will be eligible for benefits through the state or local educational agencies. The 1997 amendments to IDEA speculate that it is unlawful to use IDEA funds to pay for services, such as instrumental assessment for the diagnosis of dysphagia that would have been covered by other sources, such as insurance, if the federal funds were not available. This is the foundational argument for using Medicare or Medicaid funds to support items, such as instrumental assessment, that are part of the student's Individualized Education Plan (IEP). Many students who qualify for dysphagia services will also have concomitant medical conditions that qualify them for either Medicare or Medicaid coverage. The student's insurance plan, whether public or private, should be the payer of first resort for instrumental assessment (Power-deFur & Alley, 2008).

Conclusion

The coordination between respiratory and swallowing physiology is an intricate and delicate interplay. The two actions, breathing and swallowing, utilize many of the same anatomical features to accomplish divergent goals. Students with dysphagia will frequently present with signs and symptoms of aspiration as a result of dysphagia. Aspiration can lead to significant co-morbidity and mortality in students with dysphagia. Therefore, it is necessary to accurately identify the physiologic cause of the student's dysphagia and provide effective intervention. Accurate identification and aggressive treatment can be accomplished with the help of instrumental assessment to visualize the swallowing problems and provide information on the efficacy of chosen interventions. Speech-language pathologists within the school system who provide dysphagia services must recognize signs and symptoms of swallowing impairment and know when and how to refer for instrumental assessment. The key points discussed in this chapter provide the school speech-language pathologist with the fundamental knowledge necessary to understand the components of respiration and swallowing and when and how to make appropriate referrals for instrumental assessment of pediatric dysphagia.

References

Arvedson, J. C. (2008). Assessment of pediatric dysphagia and feeding disorders: Clinical and instrumental approaches. *Developmental Disabilities Research Reviews, 14*(2), 118–127. doi:10.1002/ddrr.17

Ball, J. W., Bindler, R. C., & Cowen, K. J. (2010). Alterations in respiratory function. *Child health nursing: Partnering with children and families* (2nd ed., pp. 838–906). Upper Saddle River, NJ: Pearson Education.

Benson, J. E., & Lefton-Greif, M. A. (1994). Videofluoroscopy of swallowing in pediatric patients: A component of the total feeding evaluation. In D. N. Tuchman & R. S. Walter (Eds.), *Disorders of feeding and swallowing in infants and children: pathophysiology, diagnosis, and treatment* (1st ed., pp. 187–200). San Diego, CA: Singular.

Bosma, J., Donner, M., Tanaka, E., & Robertson, D. (1986). Anatomy of the pharynx, pertinent to swallowing. *Dysphagia (0179051X), 1*(1), 23.

Bosma, J. F. (1972). Form and function in the infant's mouth and pharynx. In J. F. Bosma (Ed.), *Oral sensation and perception: The mouth of the infant* (pp. 3–29). Springfield, IL: Charles C. Thomas.

Bosma, J. F., & Showacre, J. (1975). *Symposium on development of upper respiratory anatomy and function: Implications for sudden infant death syndrome.* Baltimore, MD: National Institutes of Health.

Brodsky, L., & Arvesdson, J. C. (2002). Anatomy, embryology, physiology, and normal development. In J. C. Arvedson & L. Brodsky (Eds.), *Pediatric swallowing and feeding: Assessment and management* (2nd ed.). Baltimore, MD: Delmar.

Cavataio, F., & Guandalini, S. (2005). Gastroesophageal reflux. In S. Guandalini (Ed.), *Essential pediatric gastroenterology, hepatology, and nutrition* (pp. 175–173). United States: McGraw-Hill Professional.

Crelin, E. S. (1973). *Functional anatomy of the newborn.* New Haven, CT: Yale University Press.

de Benedictis, F. M., Carnielli, V. P., & de Benedictis, D. (2009). Aspiration lung disease. *Pediatric Clinics of North America, 56*(1), 173–190, xi. doi:10.1016/j.pcl.2008.10.013

Dodds, W. J. (1989). The philosophy of swallowing. *Dysphagia, 3*(4), 171–178.

Dodds, W. J., Steward, E. T., & Logemann, J. A. (1990). Physiology and radiology of the normal oral and pharyngeal phases of swallowing *American Journal of Radiology, 154,* 953–963.

Kahane, J. C. (1982). Growth of the human prepubertal and pubertal larynx. *Journal of Speech, Language, and Hearing Research, 25*(3), 446–455.

Kelly, B. N., Huckabee, M. L., Jones, R. D., & Frampton, C. M. (2007). The first year of human life: Coordinating respiration and nutritive swallowing. *Dysphagia, 22*(1), 37–43. doi:10.1007/s00455-006-9038-3

Klahn, M. S., & Perlman, A. L. (1999). Temporal and durational patterns associating respiration and swallowing. *Dysphagia, 14*(3), 131–138.

Kramer, S. S., & Eicher, P. M. (1993). The evaluation of pediatric feeding abnormalities. *Dysphagia, 8*(3), 215–224.

Laitman, J. T., & Reidenberg, J. S. (1993). Specializations of the human upper respiratory and upper digestive systems as seen through comparative and developmental anatomy. *Dysphagia, 8*(4), 318–325.

Leder, S. B., & Karas, D. E. (2000). Fiberoptic endoscopic evaluation of swallowing in the pediatric population. *Laryngoscope, 110*(7), 1132–1136. doi:10.1097/00005537-200007000-00012

Lefton-Greif, M. A. (2008). Pediatric dysphagia. *Physical Medicine and Rehabilitation Clinics of North America, 19*(4), 837–851, ix. doi:10.1016/j.pmr.2008.05.007

Lefton-Greif, M. A., & McGrath-Morrow, S. A. (2007). Deglutition and respiration: development, coordination, and practical implications. *Seminars in Speech and Language, 28*(3), 166–179. doi:10.1055/s-2007-984723

Logemann, J. A. (1998). *Evaluation and treatment of swallowing disorders.* Austin, TX: Pro-Ed.

Marieb, E. N. (1995). The respiratory system. *Human anatomy and physiology* (3rd ed., pp. 743–787). Redwood City, CA: Benjamin Cummings.

Morris, S. E., & Klein, M. D. (2000). Normal Development of Feeding Skills. In S. E. Morris & M. D. Klein (Eds.), *Pre-feeding skills, second edition: A comprehensive resource for mealtime development* (pp. 59–95). Austin, TX: Pro-Ed.

Newman, L. A. (2000). Optimal care patterns in pediatric patients with dysphagia. *Seminars in Speech and Language, 21*(4), 281–291.

Newman, L. A. (2001). Anatomy and phsyiology of the infant swallow. *SIG 13 Perspectives on Swallowing and Swallowing Disorders (Dysphagia), 10,* 3–4. doi:10.1044/sasd10.1.3

Power-deFur, L., & Alley, N. S. (2008). Legal and financial issues associated with providing services in schools to children with swallowing and feeding disorders. *Language, Speech, and Hearing Services in Schools, 39*(2), 160–166. doi:10.1044/0161-1461(2008/016)

Preiksaitis, H. G., Mayrand, S., Robins, K., & Diamant, N. E. (1992). Coordination of respiration and swallowing: Effect of bolus volume in normal adults. *American Journal of Physiology, 263*(3 Pt. 2), R624–R630.

Ramsey, G. H., Watson, J. S., Gramiak, R., & Weinberg, S. A. (1955). Cinefluorographic analysis of the mechanism of swallowing. *Radiology, 64*(4), 498–518. doi:10.1148/64.4.498

Rees, C. J. (2006). Flexible endoscopic evaluation of swallowing with sensory testing. *Current Opinion in Otolaryngology and Head and Neck Surgery, 14*(6), 425–430. doi:10.1097/MOO.0b013e328010ba88

Rommel, N., De Meyer, A. M., Feenstra, L., & Veereman-Wauters, G. (2003). The complexity of feeding problems in 700 infants and young children presenting to a tertiary care institution. *Journal of Pediatric Gastroenterology and Nutrition, 37*(1), 75–84.

Tabaee, A., Johnson, P. E., Gartner, C. J., Kalwerisky, K., Desloge, R. B., & Stewart, M. G. (2006). Patient-controlled comparison of flexible endoscopic evaluation of swallowing with sensory testing (FEESST) and videofluoroscopy. *Laryngoscope, 116*(5), 821–825. doi:10.1097/01.mlg.0000214670.40604.45

Thompson, D. M. (2003). Laryngopharyngeal sensory testing and assessment of airway protection in pediatric patients. *The American Journal of Medicine, 115*(3), 166–168.

Tuchman, D. N. (1988). Dysfunctional swallowing in the pediatric patient: Clinical considerations. *Dysphagia, 2*(4), 203–208.

Tuchman, D. N. (1994). Physiology of the Swallowing Apparatus. In D. N. Tuchman & R. S. Walter (Eds.), *Disorders of feeding and swallowing in infants and children: Pathophysiology, diagnosis, and treatment* (pp. 1–25). San Diego, CA: Singular.

Turnbull, H., & Turnbull, A. (1997). *Free appropriate public education: The law and children with disabilities* Denver, CO: Love Publishing.

Tutor, J. D., & Gosa, M. M. (2012). Dysphagia and aspiration in children. *Pediatric Pulmonology, 47*(4), 321–337. doi:10.1002/ppul.21576

Willging, J. P., & Thompson, D. M. (2005). Pediatric FEESST: Fiberoptic endoscopic evaluation of swallowing with sensory testing. *Current Gastroenterology Reports, 7*(3), 240–243.

Zemlin, W. R. (1998). *Speech and hearing science: Anatomy and physiology.* Englewood Cliffs, NJ: Prentice-Hall.

5

Management of Swallowing and Feeding in the Schools: Preschool Through 12th Grade

Emily M. Homer

Managing Swallowing and Feeding: Getting Started

Initially when a school district begins addressing swallowing and feeding, they focus on the safety of students during mealtimes. Once a school team has evaluated a student, written a swallowing and feeding plan, and trained the classroom staff to safely feed the child at school, intervention should be considered as part of the management of the disorder. There are different levels of management that will take place depending on the type and severity of the swallowing and feeding disorder. This chapter focuses on how a district can address the management and treatment of swallowing and feeding disorders once safety has been established. Information on setting up a proactive precaution program called Feeding All Students Safely (FASS) is also included, which works with classroom staff to raise awareness of feeding safety at school for all students.

Levels of Management

The types and severity of swallowing and feeding disorders that a school team will address is almost unlimited. It may be helpful to divide the treatment into levels of management. There are four levels of management that the school team needs to address with students that have been identified with a swallowing disorder. In addition, Chapter 6 has intervention tiers as a management model that offers information on working with children who exhibit behavioral feeding disorders. The four levels of management are as follows: collaborative consultation for all students, direct therapeutic intervention to improve oral phase dysphagia, intervention with students with progressive disorders or who are medically fragile, and transition to or from tube feeding (Table 5–1). Following is an explanation of each level of management, including a description of what it is, which students are involved, and how it can be implemented in the school program.

Level 1: Collaborative Consultation

Consultation involves working directly with the classroom staff and parents to address the student's swallowing and feeding issues. Consultation is part of every child's swallowing and feeding program and is indicated when a student needs ongoing environmental support to be successful. In the case of swallowing and feeding, there are many team members who work with the student and each one has an area of expertise. Collaborative consultation is an interactive process that enables partnerships of people with diverse expertise to generate creative solutions to mutually defined problems (Idol, Paolucci-Whitcomb, & Nevin, 1995). Each swallowing and feeding team member will need

Table 5–1. Levels of Management of Swallowing and Feeding Services in the Schools

Level 1 Collaborative Consultation	Level 2 Direct Therapeutic Intervention
All students followed by the swallowing and feeding team are monitored on the implementation of the swallowing and feeding plan. Ongoing consultation services are provided to classroom staff through information gathering, sharing information (education, demonstration and modeling), team coordination, providing feedback, and conflict resolution.	Oral motor treatments are done to improve oral preparatory and oral transit phases. Parents and school staff are trained, exercises are specific to the child's weaknesses, exercises are done frequently and repeatedly with fidelity, and data are taken to drive the treatment plan.
Level 3 Intervention With the Student with Progressive Disorders or Medically Fragile	Level 4 Transition to or From Tube Feeding
School team works closely with parents/guardians and physicians to monitor and adjust to changes. Medical and school team collaboration is essential. Nurse is a major team member when working with a progressive disorder.	School team shares information regarding swallowing and feeding status with parents/guardians and physicians and works closely with them to make the transition.

to consult with the other members to ensure that all areas of the student's swallowing and feeding program are successfully implemented.

What Is a Consultant?

A consultant is a professional with the knowledge and skills to mobilize other professionals in the treatment or handling of specific and mutually defined problems. A consultant serves as a resource for the professionals who actually deal with the problems. A consultant gives professional advice or services based on their knowledge on the subject matter (Merriam-Webster Dictionary, n.d.). They offer information to the teachers, paraprofessionals, and parents/guardians who are responsible for the feeding and nutritional intake of the student. To be an effective consultant it is important to understand the importance of having a positive, helpful attitude. The SLP or other professional relays a desire to help and to work together for the benefit of the student. All members of the team have something to offer and their input should not only be recognized but valued.

The Process of Consultation

There are five steps in the process of providing consultative services to those involved in serving students with swallowing and feeding disorders. This process applies to all swallowing and feeding team members including SLP, OT, PT, parent/guardian, classroom teacher, and paraprofessional. Each of the following five steps will be discussed: Step 1: Gathering Information, Step 2: Sharing Information, Step 3: Coordinating the Team, Step 4: Giving Feedback, and Step 5: Resolving Conflicts (Table 5–2).

Step 1: Gathering Information: Monitoring

The primary method of gathering information is through the process of monitoring. It is part of collaboration. Monitoring occurs when the student is observed during a mealtime on the implementation of his or her swallowing and feeding plan. Monitoring is done to ensure that the plan is being implemented correctly and to determine if changes are indicated based on the information gathered.

Monitoring includes observing the staff and providing intervention following the recommendations on the swallowing and feeding plan. During monitoring, the case manager modifies any interventions being implemented or equipment that is needed, documents the student's current feeding status, and researches solutions to complications in the feeding process. It is the case manager's responsibility to observe the student eating in a vari-

Table 5–2. Five Steps in a Collaborative Consultative Level of Treatment for Swallowing and Feeding Disorders in the Schools

Step 1: Monitoring the implementation of the swallowing and feeding plan
- Observation of feeding
- Positioning
- Food preparation
- Feeding equipment
- Food presentation

Step 2: Sharing information with swallowing and feeding team members
- Education on the who and what of a swallowing and feeding disorder
- Training on the swallowing and feeding plan
- Training on precautions
- Training on liquid and food alteration

Step 3: Coordinating swallowing and feeding team members
- Keeping team members informed of student's feeding status
- Facilitating a collaborative atmosphere

Step 4: Using feedback as part of consultative process
- Reinforcing what is being done well
- Relaying an attitude of helpfulness
- Informing feeders of what is working and what needs attention

Step 5: Resolving conflicts throughout the process
- Ensure that adequate training has occurred
- Follow up with information sharing and feedback
- Consult with classroom teacher regarding compliance
- If not responsive to the concerns, consult with principal
- If not responsive to the concerns, consult with supervisor

ety of settings at school, including the cafeteria and the classroom during snack. The swallowing and feeding plan is reviewed on a regular basis and changed as needed.

Monitoring: Determining the Amount and Type of Intervention. Once the swallowing and feeding plan has been established it is necessary for the case manager to set up a schedule for monitoring both the student and the classroom staff to ensure that the plan is being followed correctly and that there have not been changes in the student's feeding status since the plan was written. The amount of direct observation varies by student with some needing to be monitored weekly and others only needing monthly. The SLP determines the level of monitoring each student with swallowing and feeding disorders will need. This determination is based on the severity of the student's swallowing and feeding issues, the student's medical condition, the nature of the disorder, the competency of the classroom staff, and the case manager's personal professional comfort level with what is occurring in the cafeteria or classroom during mealtimes. Monitoring is structured around the implementation of the swallowing and feeding plan and the periodic adjustments that may need to be made.

The Process of Monitoring. Observation is probably the most common form of monitoring; however, there are other forms of monitoring that provide important information. Activities included in the monitoring process are:

- Observing the student feeding in several settings (example: cafeteria, snack time), looking at all areas of the plan including positioning, food preparation, food consistency, feeding techniques, and precautions.
- Documenting successful implementation of the plan in ensuring the safety of the student during meals, and if not successfully implemented, adjusting and modifying the swallowing and feeding plan and retraining the classroom staff.
- Informing the classroom staff of signs and symptoms that may indicate that the plan is not effective or that the student's swallowing and feeding skills are changing.
- Listening to the classroom staff and asking them to share their observations and concerns.

Examples of Monitoring Schedules. The following are examples of how SLPs in the schools schedule the monitoring of swallowing and feeding students:

Student Profile:
Importance of Ongoing Monitoring

Jacob was a high school student with cerebral palsy who had been followed by the swallowing and feeding team for years. Through the years, Jacob's plans were slightly tweaked but were basically the same. His condition did not change much. The swallowing and feeding case manager monitored Jacob monthly by interviewing classroom staff and parents and observing him eating at school. During his second year in high school, he began having frequent upper respiratory infections, although there were no signs or symptoms of aspiration. The case manager was concerned when this was reported and confirmed it with the parent. An interdisciplinary observation was set up with the SLP, OT, nurse, teacher, and parent participating. The nurse listened to Jacob's lungs prior to introducing any food or liquid. The lungs sounded clear. The student, who was on a puree diet, was given a small spoonful of applesauce and appeared to handle it. Another small spoonful was presented and the nurse listened to his lungs again. This time there was crackling, the lungs no longer sounded clear, and the observation was stopped. Jacob was referred for an MBSS and it was determined that he was silently aspirating on thin liquids and thin puree. His swallowing and feeding plan was adapted to specify thick puree and honey thick liquids only. Jacob ate safely at school for approximately 1 year and then was recommended by his physician for PEG tube feeding.

Example 1: The case manager observes the student in the cafeteria at lunch one time per week. During this weekly observation the SLP records how the student is responding to the plan and if it is accomplishing the goal of safe, efficient feeding. The observation is recorded on the therapy documentation log for the student and information and/or suggestions are shared with the classroom staff. The classroom staff reports to the case manager problems that they encounter. The parents/guardians receive weekly feedback regarding the student's feeding.

Example 2: The case manager consults monthly with the teacher, depending on the student, to get feedback on how the student is doing with the swallowing and feeding plan and to make adjustments if indicated. The case manager may do a direct observation of the child feeding once a month.

Example 3: In another scenario the SLP eats lunch monthly with the student to determine if the plan is appropriate and if changes need to be made. Consultation with classroom staff occurs as needed.

Each student is unique and each case may be managed in a slightly different manner depending on the student's swallowing and feeding disorder as well as the skills of the classroom staff. The SLP will be able to determine the level of monitoring that is necessary for each student and his or her comfort level with the student's feeding activities at school.

Monitoring the Implementation of the Swallowing and Feeding Plan. Most monitoring activities will be on the implementation of the swallowing and feeding plan. Each area of the plan is discussed.

Monitoring Positioning During Meals. Correct positioning can make the difference between a child who is fed safely and one who is at risk for aspiration. Physical and occupational therapists should be involved when determining appropriate positioning during meals. Positioning can be important for both ambulatory and non-ambulatory students, and there is not one position that is safe for every child when eating and drinking. The physical therapist on the team uses various methods of positioning to ensure safety during eating for each individual student. When eating at tables or in the cafeteria, students should be supported in their chairs and have their feet firmly placed on the floor. Once the best position has been identified and the classroom staff has been trained on how to place the student in the correct position for meals, the case manager observes the student's positioning on a regular basis during meals as part of monitoring management.

Monitoring Food Preparation. The staff members responsible for food preparation need to be trained to modify the student's recommended diet to the appropriate texture as instructed by the feeding plan. Once the classroom staff is trained on how to prepare the consistency of the food, the case manager will periodically observe the food preparation process to ensure that the correct foods are being placed on the tray and are being altered according to the plan.

Monitoring Feeding Equipment. Use of proper equipment is also important to the success of a student during feeding. Equipment can include suction bowls, modified spoons, modified cups, and more. The type of equipment that helps a child become successful during mealtime varies from student to student. Typically the OT will work with the student to determine the equipment that is most effective. It is suggested that spoons, cups, bowls, and other equipment be used on a trial basis until proven successful for the student. The SLP and OT monitor the effectiveness of special equipment and how it is being used.

Monitoring Correct Food Presentation. The student's swallowing and feeding plan includes directions on how food should be presented to the student. This may include bite size, where to place the food in the child's mouth, or pacing the food intake. It is important to monitor food presentation when a student's swallowing and feeding plan indicates that the child's meal is modified. Overstuffing is the most common symptom that needs to be addressed and monitored during meals. As a result of overstuffing, it may be important to adjust the amount of food available to a student by limiting what is presented on the tray and adding food as the meal progresses. Other students may need to see everything that they are expected to eat during that meal in their bowl or tray so they can know when they have completed their meal. Directions on how to present food to the student should be specific and detailed in the swallowing and feeding plan and frequently monitored.

Step 2: Sharing Information With Team Members

The SLP, OT, PT, and nurse have knowledge about swallowing and feeding disorders that when shared allows the service providers to be more proficient and competent feeding children. Sharing information may be done through direct instruction or through modeling and demonstration.

Instruction: Educating Personnel on the Disorder. Many school system employees and parents/guardians may not know or understand swallowing and feeding disorders. In many cases, they may not have ever heard of dysphagia or understand its risks. The case manager and other school team members serve as consultants, educating staff members and parents on swallowing and feeding disorders. The SLP can provide the teacher, parents/guardians, principal, or other team member with articles and references that inform them of the disorder. The Who and What of Swallowing and Feeding Disorders in the Schools (Dysphagia) Summary Sheet 1 (see Chapter 1) has information on the following:

- What is a swallowing and feeding disorder?
- Who is at risk for a swallowing and feeding disorders?
- What are some of the signs and symptoms of a swallowing and feeding disorder?
- What are the complications of a swallowing and feeding disorder?

This summary sheet is a quick and useful way to educate others on swallowing and feeding disorders. The American Speech-Language-Hearing Association and the American Occupational Therapy Association also have information online that may be distributed to parents/guardians and others.

Instruction: Training the School Staff on the Swallowing and Feeding Plan. Prior to setting up a monitoring schedule it is essential to train the classroom staff and parents/guardians on the recommendations of the swallowing and feeding plan. The speech-language pathologist and school team can create a well-thought-out swallowing and feeding plan for a student; however, if the staff that feeds the student on a regular basis is trained ineffectively, or not trained at all, the plan may not be implemented with fidelity. The SLP or case manager should be present during meals until confident that the classroom staff has been thoroughly trained and can safely feed the student. Some students with complex feeding issues are difficult to feed and may require repetition and practice during training to help the staff feel more confident in their ability to feed the student safely.

Demonstrating and modeling how a student should be fed according to the plan is part of the training process. The classroom staff observes the case manager feeding the student and can ask questions and get clarification. For example, the SLP goes into the cafeteria and demonstrates for the classroom staff the position the student should be in for feeding, the amount of food per spoon, and the cueing to swallow twice before presenting another spoon of food. Modeling and demonstrating the techniques for the classroom staff, and in many cases the parents, is an effective way to ensure that they understand exactly how the student should be fed. Parents/guardians may also demonstrate for the classroom staff how they feed their child at home. In most cases parents/guardians have figured out how to safely feed their child at home. The team often benefits from the parent's demonstration. It can also be an opportunity for the case manager to discuss with the parents/guardians other strategies that may make the student safer or more efficient during mealtimes.

Instruction: Training the Classroom Staff on Precautions. When training classroom staff on how to feed a student with swallowing and feeding concerns, it is important to discuss possible precautions. Precautions can include having the student sit upright for a period of time following a meal, bite to drink ratio, and swallow to food presentation ratio. Precautions should be specific and detailed and based on the swallowing and feeding plan. If the child should be given sips of drink after every two bites of food it should be written that way in the plan. These plans are written for teachers and paraprofessionals, not SLPs. The plan should be specific enough that if a substitute feeder comes into the room, he or she would understand the swallowing and feeding plan, and be able to feed the student safely.

Instruction: Training Staff on Liquid and Food Alteration. The case manager, usually the SLP or OT, works with the classroom staff on how to prepare the recommended consistency for liquids and foods in the child's swallowing and feeding plan. For example, if the diet orders indicate a puree consistency, the case manager should work with the teacher and paraprofessional until there is an agreement on the puree consistency. It takes practice to get the consistency of the food the same over time. Similarly, it can be difficult to prepare nectar thick juice or other drinks the same every day. Once the staff has been trained to alter the student's meals, the case manager should continue to work with the classroom staff and monitor liquid and food consistency and preparation.

Step 3: Coordinating the Efforts of the Swallowing and Feeding Team Members

Working as a team is always a challenge and requires someone who is able to coordinate the efforts of all of the professionals and the parents/guardians. The case manager is responsible for keeping team members updated on the student's status and to facilitate working together in a collaborative atmosphere. Part of the consultative process with swallowing and feeding is for the SLP or case manager to relay to other team members the mutual goals of the team and establish a method for team members to share solutions to achieving the goals. This could include regularly scheduled meetings, e-mail correspondence, conference calls, or weekly/monthly updates in a log or notebook.

Step 4: Using Feedback as Part of the Consultative Process

Feedback is an essential part of a consultant's job and should be approached with preparation of what will be addressed, how it will be presented, and what the potential outcome should be. In order for the classroom staff to feed the student safely according to the swallowing and feeding plan, the case manager will provide them with constructive and descriptive feedback. They need to know exactly what they are doing correctly and what they need to adjust. When an SLP or other professional goes into a cafeteria or classroom to observe a student eating it is important that the observer reinforces what is being done well and then directs and instructs on what needs to be done differently. Whenever possible, begin with a positive statement and relay an attitude of helpfulness. For example: "I am here to see how you are doing. How is it going? The consistency of the food that you are preparing looks great. What's not working? It looks like he's having some trouble with the amount of food being presented, let's try giving him half that amount." This dialogue is an example of a consultation where the SLP first gathers information from the feeder and then offers help. It is done in a nonthreatening manner and relays an interest in assisting rather than judging. When giving feedback to teachers and paraprofessionals it is helpful for them to know directly and descriptively what is being done well and what needs some attention. The case manager should follow up with a written summary of the observation and suggestions.

Step 5: Resolving Conflicts

There may be situations where the classroom staff does not follow the recommendations on the swallowing and feeding plan. If the case manager has documented that training was done, there has been ongoing consultation, that the staff was redirected on how to correctly feed the student, and the problem continues then it may be necessary to involve administration. The suggested process for addressing the situation where a paraprofessional is either refusing to follow the swallowing and feeding plan or is not able to follow it is as follows:

- Always talk to the paraprofessional directly explaining to them the importance of following the plan.
- If the issue is not resolved, talk privately to the classroom teacher and seek his or her assistance in getting the paraprofessional to comply or in assigning a different feeder to the student.
- If the teacher does not cooperate, inform them that because of the seriousness of this issue, you must inform the principal of their failure to follow the student's feeding plan thus putting the child at risk.

- Speak to the principal about the concerns. Inform him or her of what you have done so far, and ask for assistance in accomplishing compliance.
- If the principal does not enforce compliance, then contact the supervisor. At this level the case manager may need to educate the supervisor on the disorder and why compliance is so important.

In most cases paraprofessionals and/or teachers are efficient and conscientious when feeding students according to their swallowing and feeding plan, but there are situations where they do not follow the procedure and therefore the consultant will need to follow up on how to enforce compliance.

Level 2: Direct Therapeutic Intervention to Improve Oral Phase Dysphagia

Children with swallowing and feeding disorders in the school setting are often delayed in their oral motor development and some have disorders that compromise the structure and function of the oral motor mechanism. When working with children with oral dysphagia, therapy focuses on helping students progress in their development or acquisition of oral motor skills as well as maximize the function of the skills that they currently have developed. According to Angell, Bailey, Nicholson, and Stoner (2009), there is no single type of intervention that will be effective with all children with swallowing and feeding disorders. The effectiveness of therapeutic intervention is tied to the needs of the child and the student's unique situations.

Oral Motor Therapy Evidence

Research available neither proves that oral motor therapy for children with swallowing and feeding disorders works nor doesn't work. According to the Royal College of Speech and Language Therapists clinical guidelines (Taylor-Goh, 2005), which contained at least one controlled clinical study, "The Speech

& Language Therapist will provide therapy to maintain and/or improve oromotor function, which will be within agreed optimal time frames. This may include range of motion, chewing and swallowing exercises, and thermal and tactile stimulation."

A review of studies that examined oral sensorimotor treatment or a lip strengthening program stated that "there is currently not enough high-quality evidence from randomized controlled trials to provide conclusive results about the effectiveness of any particular type of therapy . . . no clear guidelines or recommendations for clinical practice with this population of children can be made until higher-quality evidence has been generated" (Morgan, Dodrill, & Ward, 2012). Other studies and reviews came to similar conclusions that there was not sufficient evidence to determine the effectiveness of oral motor exercises on swallowing and feeding (Arvedson, Clark, Lazarus, Schooling, & Frymark, 2010; Davies, 2003; Snider, Majnemer, & Darsaklis, 2011; Walshe, Smith, & Pennington, 2012).

While the research is limited and inconclusive, there seems to be strong clinical expertise/expert opinion supporting the use of oral motor exercises to address oral phase dysphagia. According to Bahr (2008), recent presentations and articles on oral motor treatment have been narrowly defined and equated with nonspeech oral exercise, which has caused significant confusion and misunderstanding within the field.

Therapists may need to rely on a combination of the limited research available, the clinical expertise that is recorded in the literature and their own experiences, knowledge, and data on what is effective. Effectiveness will depend on many factors including the nature of the student's disorder, the limitations of the student's neuromuscular condition, and the individual response to treatment.

Definition of Oral Motor Function and Treatment

For the purpose of this chapter, the following definitions are used to describe oral motor function and oral motor treatment:

Oral motor function is fine motor function of the oral mechanism (i.e., jaw, tongue, lips, and cheeks) for the purposes of eating, drinking, speaking, and other mouth activities (Bahr, 2008).

Oral motor treatment addresses sensory processing as well as dissociation, grading, direction, timing, and coordination of mouth movement for eating, drinking, speaking, and other mouth activities. The speech-language pathologist focuses treatment on eating, drinking, and speaking (Bahr, 2008).

Treatment Options With Oral Phase Dysphagia in the Schools

Children with oral phase dysphagia have difficulty chewing and forming a bolus. Students may benefit from a program that works to improve chewing and swallowing, helps to maintain oral motor functioning to prevent a decrease in functioning level, and moves a student to progress towards a more normalized diet. The program should be intensive and systematic. Data should be collected frequently to determine its effectiveness. If the student is not progressing or is not responding to the oral motor therapy, the exercises should be stopped and a different approach should be used. Sheppard (2005) suggests five basic treatment principles essential for habilitation or rehabilitation of motor disorders:

1. Therapy strategies used address the specific neuromuscular impairments that are affecting the student's functioning.
2. Student sits upright with adequate postural support and stability.
3. Therapy strategies are applied immediately before the student eats or drinks.
4. Oral motor skills are trained in the order that they normally develop.
5. Demands of the treatment tasks are increased and facilitation strategies are reduced in response to the student's progress.

Oral Motor Assessment

Before beginning an oral motor treatment program the SLP should evaluate the student's oral motor skills. There are two different methods of assessing oral motor functioning:

- Active: which is done during functional tasks with feeding trials, and/or imitation tasks
- Facilitated/passive: muscle movement is manipulated and scored on the amount of movement per muscle group (Edwards, Gould, Mayfield, & Simon, 2013)

There are commercially produced pediatric oral motor and feeding assessments that can be used to determine a student's neuromuscular impairments, oral motor function, and oral motor movements during feeding. A thorough oral motor assessment will help to identify the source of the student's difficulties and to design a treatment plan.

Oral Motor Treatments

When working on any oral motor skill, exercises chosen should be based on clinically observed deficits in the child. Edwards et al., (2013) recommend that SLPs treating pediatric oral motor skills target normal movement patterns by inhibiting abnormal and/or compensatory movements. Treatments should target specific skills that are functional and meaningful such as spoon-feeding, biting, chewing, cup drinking, and straw drinking.

Positioning is important when addressing oral motor treatments designed to improve feeding skills. Postural stability alignment and control must be considered for normal movement patterns to develop and is required to support functional movement for feeding. Other strategies may include thickening liquids to control spillage until the student's skills develop, placing foods that are safe for the student directly on the molars and using controlled placement of puree foods in the student's mouth to work on crossing the midline with the tongue (Gisel, 1994). It is important to note that oral exercises alone may not improve feeding abilities but can be effective as part of an entire therapy protocol. When doing oral motor treatment, consistency and repetition is important. Any change in motor skills should do the following: build in overload capacity and progression, focus on speed and endurance and on movements related to bolus management and swallowing (Mansolillo, 2015).

Therapist Manipulated Exercises. Mechanical muscle response exercises provide assisted movement to activate muscle contraction and to provide movement against resistance to build strength. This method includes exercises that work on lips, cheeks, jaw, and tongue (Beckman, Neal, Phirsichbaum, Stratton, Taylor, & Ratusnik, 2004). These may be useful for children who do not have the cognitive ability to perform therapist-directed exercises. Clinically, these exercises help to desensitize orally defensive children and improve lateralization.

Oral Massage, Oral Stimulation, and Vibration to Facilitate Movement. Many students at a young age exhibit high, low, or fluctuating tone in the oral cavity. Weaknesses in lip closure may be due to low tone or motor weakness. According to Diane Bahr (2001), oral massage may be used to increase oral awareness, decrease tonic bite; decrease hyperactive gag reflex, and decrease tooth grinding. It can also be used for students with tone issues, as well as with students with strength and coordination concerns. Edwards et al. (2013) suggest that massage and stretching exercises may be successful in promoting awareness of oromotor structures, facilitating symmetrical movement as level of food challenge is gradually increased, and improving feeding.

Therapists report that using the Z-vibe or other vibrating tools with these students helps to facilitate movement. Low tone children seem more responsive when vibration is also used in conjunction with oral massage. A slow deep massage may be used to facilitate muscle relaxation.

Vibration and oral stimulation is used to desensitize and "wake up" the muscles of the oral mechanism. Vibration can be used on the tongue, cheeks, and inside and outside of the mouth. Vibration can be accomplished by using mouth massagers and vibrators, as well as a vibrating toothbrush. They may be used to increase lip closure, cheek strength, lip strength and seal, lip awareness, tongue lateralization, and jaw stability. Vibrators should never be used with children who have a history of seizures or who are high risk for a seizure disorder.

Jaw Work. Improving jaw function can affect the overall ability to bite, chew, and to form a bolus. Exercises directed toward jaw stability, strength, and function are used to encourage and practice biting and chewing to prepare a student for new food textures. Chewy tubes and other products have been used in therapy to strengthen jaw movement and as a precursor to chewing food. The chewy tube or other jaw exerciser is placed on the back molar, noting that the jaw is aligned correctly, and then solid graded chews are done repeatedly on each side. Therapists report success in awareness of jaw action and movement as a preparation for chewing food and as a means of establishing jaw stability and strength. Oral motor tools can be dipped in yogurt or other smooth foods as a prefeeding activity.

Specificity of Training: Using Food to Target Motor Skills

Specificity of training, the specific effect of training on the muscles, is dependent on the specific stimulus (Cerny & Sapienza, 2007). Numerous studies have shown that strength gained during exercise does not readily generalize to movements unlike the exercise itself. Applying the principle of specificity, the SLP and OT should select exercises that closely match the target function. For example, if the goal is for the student to use rotary movements when chewing, then the exercise may include food placed in the back on the molars with the student directed to move it to the other side of his or her mouth. SLPs report that using real food to address tongue lateralization, and oral motor coordination is the most effective means of achieving the goal. Oral motor training goals should involve training the student as close to the desired mealtime target as possible using successive approximations. To ensure safety when working with students who are a choking risk, therapists use food wrapped in cheesecloth. The cheesecloth wrapped food is presented to the student on the molars and the student is instructed to chew. Foods that are already tolerated by the child are chosen initially when introducing this strategy.

Documentation and Data Taking

Documentation must be collected when using an oral motor treatment plan to be sure that the program is being followed and that positive changes are occurring. When developing an oral motor program for a student, baseline data should be taken at the onset of the program. The same SLP or OT should train each professional who works with the student on how to implement the program. The oral motor sequence of activities and feeding therapy strategies chosen should be done for an extensive period of time to determine if the student is responding to the therapy. All parties responsible for the treatments should be aware of what exercises are prescribed, how often each exercise should be repeated, and the response should be recorded on a documentation sheet after each session. Video recording the student prior to starting the plan and then again after 3 to 6 months of treatment will help in determining the success of the treatment program. The data will serve as a guide as to whether or not to continue the oral motor treatment plan.

Clinical Expertise

It is clear that clinically many SLPs continue to see value in oral motor treatments when properly defined, individualized based on deficiencies, and evaluated with frequent, specific data taking. Therapists see many different children with unique disorders and they need a variety of "tools" in their tool chest to design a treatment program for each child according to their specific situation. Oral motor treatments reportedly work for some children and do not appear to make a difference for others. For those who respond, they can significantly improve the child's feeding skills but should not be used when progress is not observed.

Level 3: Intervention With the Student With a Progressive Disorder or is Medically Fragile

The range of swallowing and feeding disorders in the schools is extensive and includes children who have progressive disorders and/or syndromes, which result in regression over time and children who are medically fragile. These children present a unique challenge to the swallowing and feeding team because not only does their condition change over time but they are frequently sick. Treating these students requires constant communication and collaboration with the parents/guardians and the child's physicians. Examples of progressive disorders include syndromes, diseases, and disorders such as Hunter syndrome, Batten disease, and neuromuscular atrophy.

Adjusting to Swallowing and Feeding Changes

Children with progressive disorders or who are medically fragile will need frequent and ongoing monitoring of their swallowing and feeding skills to ensure that the plan continues to be appropriate. Following each illness, the case manager should observe the student eating and make adjustments to the plan when indicated. The team needs to determine whether the way the student is being fed is contributing to his or her illness. As the feeding condition changes, difficult decisions need to be made. The swallowing and feeding team may have concerns that require difficult and complex decisions. The district team may have questions such as:

- Can the student continue to eat safely at school?
- Does the student need an alternative method of receiving nutrition?
- Is the student so sick that hospital/homebound services are indicated?

Often the progression of the disease or syndrome is slow and swallowing and feeding regression takes years to develop. School-based swallowing and feeding teams may change several times as the child moves on to higher grades. Maintaining accurate documentation of all of the evaluations, swallowing and feeding plans, and communication with parents/guardians and physicians is essential. The swallowing and feeding case manager should keep a log of all communication with the parents/guardians and physicians in the student's folder.

Team Effort

Students with progressive or terminal illnesses will require all members of the swallowing and feeding team working and communicating together to address the student's needs. It is essential that the district use its available resources including the services of a social worker or mental health provider to help the students, their parents/guardians, and classmates adjust as the disease or syndrome progresses. The principal should be informed of the student's condition and of the changes in the student's status as they occur. When a student with dysphagia returns to school following a serious illness the case manager should monitor the child to determine if swallowing and feeding skills have been affected.

The school nurse plays an important role with the student who is medically fragile or who is frequently sick. Depending on the student's condition, the nurse may need to chart health concerns at school such as suctioning, sleeping versus awake time, coughing, frequency and amount of urination. In addition, the nurse can record respiration rate, temperature, weight, and/or listen to the student's lungs for crackling indicating the possibility of aspiration. Frequently the school nurse provides physicians with information on how the student is eating and functioning at school as part of necessary ongoing communication.

Establishing an Emergency Plan at School

The school should have an emergency plan in place that outlines what conditions will necessitate the school contacting the parents/guardians or calling emergency medical services (EMS). If these issues are planned for ahead of time, it will prevent misunderstandings and confusion that can occur during an emergency situation. School staff members who work with the student should be trained on the emergency plan.

Providing Support to the Family

The families of children with a progressive disorder or who are medically fragile may need the support and understanding of school personnel. When addressing swallowing and feeding disorders with a child that may be terminal, the swallowing and feeding team members should be sensitive to the wishes and requests from the family. The team should gather and provide helpful information to the parents.

Level 4: Transition to or From Tube Feeding

School districts educate all students including those with major medical conditions. Districts have the responsibility to provide FAPE to students, which in many cases means addressing health issues that allow students access to their curriculum. The school swallowing and feeding team provides valuable information to parents/guardians and the medical team regarding the student's feeding at school that may support either moving a student to enteral feeding or transitioning the student from tube feeding.

What Is Enteral Tube Feeding?

There are three types of tube feeding that are used most often. They are nasogastric, gastrostomy, and jejunostomy. Each of these use a high-calorie liquid food mixture containing protein, carbohydrates (sugar), fats, vitamins, and minerals that is delivered to the feeding site. These high-calorie formulas provide the nutrition the student needs on a schedule designated by the physician.

Nasogastric Tube Feeding

The nasogastric tube is inserted through the child's nostril into the pharynx, through the pharyngoesophageal segment into the esophagus. In most cases, a nasogastric tube is inserted when the condition is likely to improve and the child will return to oral feeding or will need a more permanent solution such as the percutaneous endoscopic gastrostomy (PEG) tube. The movements and activities of children can move the tube out of place presenting an aspiration risk. The American Association of Critical Care Nurses (Bourgault, Heath, Hooper, Sole, & Nesmith,,

2015) recommend that placement of the nasogastric tube be assessed at 4-hour intervals. A nurse or medical staff must do this assessment and therefore nasogastric tube feeding is extremely difficult in the school setting.

Percutaneous Endoscopic Gastrostomy (PEG) Tube Feeding

The most common form of tube feeding in the schools is the PEG tube also referred to as G-tube. The PEG tube is a gastrostomy tube that is placed in the stomach and nutrition is received directly into the stomach. Some students receive their tube feeding on a typical feeding schedule whereas others are on a slow continuous feed. The school nurse will train classroom staff on how to feed the student at school. In school districts there are students with disorders such as severe cerebral palsy whose oral mechanism is so compromised that they are unable to take food orally in spite of having an adequate pharyngeal swallow. These students may have a PEG tube but can continue to be fed orally for pleasure. Other students are at such a high risk for aspiration that they cannot receive any food orally.

Jejunostomy Tube Feeding

The jejunostomy or J-tube is inserted directly into the student's small intestine when the stomach is not working. This tube is used less often but has the same considerations as the PEG in relation to oral feeding and training.

When Does a Person Need Enteral Feeding?

There are three reasons why a physician prescribes tube feeding for a child. The first reason is when a child is unable to sustain nutrition orally but has a safe pharyngeal swallow. This condition is called "failure to thrive" and the student may or may not be able to eventually return to oral feeding. Nutrition is received through a PEG tube until their weight is managed and they are able to obtain sufficient calories orally. Tube feeding may occur for months or years depending on the situation. The second situation where tube feeding may be recommended is when a child is so sick that he or she is unable to eat normally and is too fragile to risk the surgical insertion of a PEG or J-tube. Temporary, short-term nutrition is typically received through a nasogastric tube in these situations until their acute medical situation is resolved.

The final reason that a student receives enteral feeding is when there is a risk of aspiration that cannot be addressed with food alteration, positioning, or feeding strategies. These students are at such a high risk for aspirate pneumonia that they are unable to receive any nutrition or hydration, including medicine, orally (Groher & Crary, 2010).

District's Role in Moving a Student to Tube Feeding

The decision to tube feed a student rests with the parents/guardian and the medical team; however, the school team can be extremely knowledgeable about the student's feeding status and can play an important role in supporting or seeking the decision. The SLP on the school team and the school nurse together have an important role in communicating concerns to both the parents/guardians and physicians. When the school team has evidence that the student is unable to receive adequate and/or safe nutrition and hydration at school orally, they have both a legal and ethical responsibility to work with the parents/guardians and physician to ensure that the student's feeding status is addressed.

In most cases the school team shares information and works closely with the parents/guardians and physicians. The parents/guardians respect the school team's opinion and appreciate the effort the team makes in treating the child's swallowing and feeding. However, in some cases, parents refuse to consider tube feeding their child, even when recommended by the treating physician. This can put the school team in a difficult situation. As stated previously, once a student is on a public school campus the district must do everything possible to ensure that the child is safe at school and receives adequate nutrition and hydration. When a physician recommends that a child receive nothing per oral (NPO) because of a health risk and the parents refuse tube feeding, the school is unable to continue to feed the child at school. Adults in the same situation, understanding the risks involved, have the option of making a quality of life decision supported by the Patient Self-Determination Act to continue oral feeds. Parents/guardians make those decisions for children; however, regardless of the decision by the parents/guardians, and in some cases older students themselves, the school district must adhere to their responsibility to ensure that the child is safe at school and cannot feed the student at school. This can become an ethical dilemma for the school team and the district.

In the case of a child with a terminal illness, this decision making may be different and the school team may choose to follow the directives of the treating physician. Whenever there is a legal question regarding how swallowing and feeding disorders are addressed in the school setting the district should contact the school board attorney who is familiar with school law and IDEA.

Student Profile: Quality of Life

Josh is a high school student with Spinal Muscular Atrophy type II (similar to ALS). The swallowing and feeding team had followed him since he was in second grade. Through the years, Josh's swallowing and feeding plan was revised as he lost functioning. By high school, he was limited to certain foods that easily broke up and did not require much chewing. Josh was cognitively intact and enjoyed the socialization of eating. He was experiencing frequent upper respiratory infections and missed a lot of school due to pneumonia. He was referred for an MBSS. During the study, he aspirated on everything presented and the physician recommended a PEG tube for all oral intake (NPO). Josh and his mother decided that they did not want a tube and that they would make a "quality of life" decision for him to continue to eat orally. The school district, however, could not allow Josh to eat at school because he was a safety risk for aspiration. This was an extremely difficult decision for the team members who worked closely with him. He needed the socialization but could not eat at school. The decision was reached that his father would pick him up and he would eat at home. He then returned to school for his classes.

Transitioning a Student From Tube Feeding to Oral Feeding

When a student is fed by tube as a result of undernutrition and not aspiration risk, then he or she will in most cases be able to return to oral feeding. The decision to wean a student from tube feeding lies with the physician and the student's parents/guardians. The school team plays an important role in providing information on the student's oral feeding status at school. It is extremely important for the student who is tube fed as the result of failure to thrive to continue to eat orally and to be presented with a variety of food tastes and textures. The student who has received little or no foods orally is at risk for developing sensitivity to different food tastes, textures and colors and/or a behavioral feeding disorder. When a student in the school district is first prescribed enteral feeding, the school team should consult with the parents/guardians and discuss how to continue to expand the child's exposure to different foods. By continuing to feed the child orally, even in small amounts, a behavior feeding disorder may be prevented from developing.

District's Role in Transitioning to Oral Feeding

When beginning a process for weaning a child from tube feeding the school district must be sure that it is safe to begin introducing oral feeding to the student at school. This will require close collaboration with the student's medical team and parents/guardians. The school team should recognize that the district does not have total responsibility for this transition but can assist and facilitate the process during school feedings. In some cases, the medical team does not supply the parents with a plan for weaning or the parents do not understand how to do the transition and the expertise of the school team may be the parent's/guardian's only detailed, specific plan for transitioning to oral feedings.

The physician, however, may send the parents/guardians to a dietician to plan the student's nutritional transition. The district team works closely with the parents/guardians and the dietician to ensure that the student is getting adequate nutrition and hydration. A food diary is helpful in charting the types and amount of food and liquids that are offered to the student at school and the amount of food and liquids consumed by the child (see Appendix K). It is beneficial if the home and school follow the same program for introducing foods and textures. A reciprocal communication with the parents/guardians and the school team provides a smoother transition.

General Guidelines for Transitioning a Student From Tube to Oral Feeding

The process of adding different foods to a child's diet when transitioning can be similar to the one used for children with behavioral and/or sensory feeding disorders. Begin with foods that the student already eats in the same texture, and so forth, as he or she is accustomed. It may be better, depending on the student's response to the foods offered, to work on only one change at a time, such as adding a new taste (salty, sweet) or changing the texture (smooth to mixed). It may be necessary when adding different flavors to experiment with different foods to find one that the student accepts. Once they accept that food then the team can try to introduce similar foods. Some students will respond well to oral feeding and will not need to have a systematic process; however, ensuring adequate nutrition is the goal for students and the school team will support the parents/guardians in working to achieve it.

Feeding All Students Safely: Precaution Program for Students Who Are High Risk for Choking

The establishment of a swallowing and feeding team in a school district allows them to use the team member's skills and knowledge to be proactive in preventing choking accidents. Implementing a FASS program provides classroom staff members with important information on safely feeding all children with motor and/or cognitive deficits.

Who Is at Risk in the Schools for Choking?

There are two groups of students in public school districts who are high risk for choking regardless of being identified as having a swallowing and feeding disorder or not. The first group is preschool early intervention students. These students are usually between 3 to 5 years old and have some identified developmental disorder. They are often functioning significantly below their age level, placing them at risk for choking. The other group is children who have moderate to severe profound disabilities. These children have low cognitive skills and oral motor weaknesses that also make them a choking risk. Students in both of these groups are often unable to eat independently. The swallowing and feeding team already follows some of the children in these groups. By training the teachers and paraprofessionals who work in these types of classes to recognize, avoid, or alter foods that may be difficult to chew and/or swallow, the district can prevent unfortunate incidents from occurring.

FASS Program

The swallowing and feeding case manager trains the classroom staff that work with students who are preschool early intervention and/or moderate to severe profound on his or her campuses at least once a year. The training educates the classroom staff on precautions for feeding that are similar to feeding a toddler, as many of the children in these classes function like a much younger child. The training includes the following:

- Identification of foods to avoid
- Supervision requirements when children are eating.
- Structure during mealtimes
- Preparation of foods
- Restrictions when eating
- Reminders to chew
- Review of safety precautions for each student

Identification of Foods to Avoid

Some foods are very difficult for children with oral motor weaknesses and/or cognitive deficits to maneuver. Some of these foods are commonly presented in school cafeterias. Classroom staff should be able to recognize which foods would not be appropriate for each individual student in their classroom. Not all students are at the same developmental level and some will be able to handle different food items; however, some general food precautions should be utilized. The following foods, in many cases, should be avoided with children in these groups: whole grapes, nuts, marshmallows, hard candies, lollipops, gum, peanut butter, hot dogs that have not been cut lengthwise, raw fruits and vegetables (bananas and kiwi are fine), popcorn, chips, nachos, food with pits, chewy candy, caramel, stringy food, and leafy green vegetables.

Supervision Requirements When Children Are Eating

A classroom staff member should be assigned to each child when they are eating. One adult can supervise several children during mealtimes, and by designating which children each adult will be watching, the chances of a child being overlooked is reduced. This is particularly important during classroom parties, school events, and special celebrations where students are able to choose what they want to eat. Many times at these events there are chips, dips with raw vegetables, chewy treats, and other foods that may be appealing to children but may also be outside their skill level. A classroom adult will need to monitor the student's choices during these activities.

Structure During Mealtimes

All children are safer when mealtimes are structured and free from distractions. This is particularly important when the students have difficulty chewing. When eating snacks in the classroom children should be seated at a table. The atmosphere should be calm and students should have sufficient time to eat their food. There should not be other activities going on during snack or mealtimes. For example, during snack time one classroom teacher played a game with the students. While most students could handle playing the game while eating some could not. This distraction from eating put the students at a higher risk for choking.

Preparation of Foods

Some foods need to be altered in order to be safe. The classroom staff may need to cut foods into small pieces, removing seeds and pits. Vegetables should be cooked or steamed to soften their texture. Hot dogs are one of the most dangerous foods for young children especially developmentally delayed children to eat: yet they are a regular menu item in school cafeterias and at school special events. For children with oral motor weaknesses and for very young children hot dogs should be cut both lengthwise and widthwise.

Restrictions When Eating

There are some procedures that the classroom staff can do that will help students to safely swallow their food. The staff should offer students plenty of liquids during meals and snacks. Solid food and liquids, however, should be offered separately and should not be swallowed at the same time. A food to liquid ratio of one sip of liquid for every three bites may be sufficient.

When preparing a student's food, the classroom staff should consider the shape, size, and consistency of the food being offered. The amount of food offered may also need to be controlled.

Reminders to Chew

Many children in the preschool early intervention and the moderate to severe profound classes need to be reminded to chew their food completely before taking another bite. The classroom staff should be trained to regularly remind students to chew their food completely.

Review of Safety Precautions for Each Student

Each student in these classes is unique and different. The school nurse should review precautions with the classroom staff to identify safety risks when eating for each student. The nurse trains the classroom staff to recognize a child in distress and to react appropriately during a crisis. The nurse then conducts yearly review training or, on request, instruction on the Heimlich maneuver and how it should be performed on each child in the classroom

Promoting Safe Eating Habits

One of the most effective methods of teaching children to eat safely is for the teacher and classroom staff to model safe eating habits by taking small bite sizes, chewing food thoroughly before taking another bite, alternating liquids and solids, and focusing on eating and not other activities.

The FASS program provides teachers and paraprofessionals with helpful information on how to have a safe feeding environment with their students. The program encourages the swallowing and feeding team specialists to establish a working relationship with the classroom staff that encourages collaboration for the benefit of all students. The result of acting proactively is that students are safer and the risk of a choking incident is reduced.

Summary Sheet 3: Prevention of Feeding Difficulties in Students With Significant Cognitive and Motor Deficits

---

FASS: Feed All Students Safely

A Program of Prevention and Awareness

- Swallowing and feeding case manager trains teachers and paraprofessionals of preschool early intervention students and/or students with significant cognitive and motor impairments at your school on how to feed children safely.
- Teachers and paraprofessionals are in-serviced on the FASS procedure at least once during the school year.
- Follow-up visits as necessary

Swallowing and Feeding Case Manager:

_____

Contact Info: _____

_____

continues

Precautions and Preventions

- Students should always be supervised when eating.
- Students should have the muscular and developmental ability needed to chew and swallow the foods chosen. Remember, not all students will be at the same developmental level. Students with special health care needs are especially vulnerable to choking risks.
- Students should have a calm, unhurried meal and snack time.
- Students should not eat when walking or playing.
- Cut foods into small pieces, removing seeds and pits. Cook or steam vegetables to soften their texture. Cut hot dogs lengthwise and widthwise.
- Model safe eating habits by chewing food thoroughly.
- Offer plenty of liquids to children when eating, but solids and liquids should not be swallowed at the same time. Offer liquids between mouthfuls.
- Think of shape, size, consistency, and combinations of these when choosing foods.

Food Safety for Students With Significant Disabilities: Do Not Feed Students:

- Whole grapes
- Nuts
- Marshmallows
- Hard candies
- Peanut butter
- Hot dogs or meat sticks that have not been cut in half lengthwise
- Raw fruits and vegetables
- Popcorn, chips, nachos
- Food with pits such as olives
- Leafy green vegetables
- Meat that has not been cut into small pieces
- Stringy foods
- Chewy foods such as fruit snacks or caramel

References

Angell, M., Bailey, R., Nicholson, J., & Stoner, J. (2009). Family involvement in school-based dysphagia management. *Physical Disabilities: Education and Related Services, 28*(1), 6–24.

Arvedson, J., Clark, H., Lazarus, C., Schooling, T., & Frymark, T. (2010). The effects of oral-motor exercises on swallowing in children: An evidence-based systematic review. *Developmental Medicine and Child Neurology, 52*(11), 1000–1013.

Bahr, D. (2008, Nov.). *The oral motor debate: where do we go from here?* Poster session with extensive handout presented at the annual meeting of the American Speech-Language-Hearing Association, Chicago, IL.

Beckman, D., Neal, C., Phirsichbaum, J., Stratton, L., Taylor, V., & Ratusnik, D. (2004). Range of movement and strength in oral motor therapy: A retrospective study. *Florida Journal of Communication Disorders, 21*, 7–14.

Bourgault, A., Heath, J., Hooper, V., Sole, M. L., & Nesmith, E., (2015). Methods used by critical care nurses to verify feeding tube placement in clinical practice. *Critical Care Nurse, 35*(1), 1–7.

Cerny, F. J., & Sapienza, C. (2007). *Basic concepts in muscular conditioning.* ASHA convention presentation. Retrieved from http://www.asha.org/events/convention/handouts/2007/1178_sapienza_christine/

Consultant. (n.d.) In *Merriam-Webster Dictionary.com.* Retrieved April 15, 2015, from http://www.merriam-webster.com/dictionary

Davies, F. (2003). Does the end justify the means? A critique of oromotor treatment in children with cerebral palsy. *Asia Pacific Journal of Speech, Language and Hearing, 8*(2), 146–52.

Edwards, D., Gould, C., Mayfield, E., & Simon, M. (2013). *Pediatric Jaw function: Information you can chew on.* ASHA convention presentation. Retrieved from http://www.asha.org/events/convention/handouts/2013/1676-mayfield/

Gisel, E. G. (1994). Oral-motor skills following sensorimotor intervention in the moderately eating-impaired child with cerebral palsy. *Dysphagia, 9*, 180–192.

Groher, M., & Crary, M. (2010). *Dysphagia: Clinical management in adults and children* (pp. 308–320). Maryland Heights, MO: Mosby, Elsevier.

Idol, L., Paolucci-Whitcomb, P., & Nevin, A. (1995) The collaborative consultation model. *Journal of Educational and Psychological Consultation, 6*(4), 329–346, doi:10.1207/s1532768xjepc0604 3

Mansolillo, A. (2015). *Eating with ease: Managing complex feeding and swallowing problems in children.* Oral presentation to school district, Covington, LA.

Morgan, A. T., Dodrill, P., & Ward, E. C. (2012). Interventions for oropharyngeal dysphagia in children with neurological impairment. *Cochrane Database of Systematic Reviews, 10,* P.16.CD009456.

Nutrition Care. (2015). Retrieved from https://www.nutritioncare.org

Sheppard, J. J. (2005, June). The role of oral sensorimotor therapy in the treatment of pediatric dysphagia. *SIG 13 Perspectives on Swallowing and Swallowing Disorders (Dysphagia), 14,* 6–10. doi:10.1044/sasd14.2.6

Snider, L., Majnemer, A., & Darsaklis, V., (2011). Feeding interventions for children with cerebral palsy: A review of the evidence. *Physical & Occupational Therapy in Pediatrics, 31*(1), 58–77.

Taylor-Goh, S. (Ed.). (2005). *Disorders of feeding, eating, drinking & swallowing (Dysphagia), Royal College of Speech and Language Therapists Clinical Guidelines: 5.8 P.69 RCSLT Clinical Guidelines.* Bicester, UK: Speechmark.

Walshe, M., Smith, M., & Pennington, L. (2012). Interventions for drooling in children with cerebral palsy. *Cochrane Database of Systematic Reviews, 2,* 30. CD008624.

6

Working With Children With Behavioral and/or Sensorimotor Feeding Disorders

Emily M. Homer

Introduction to School-Based Behavioral Feeding Disorders

Addressing swallowing and feeding disorders in the school setting is always a challenge. Therapists in the schools often have large caseloads and increasing paperwork demands. This leaves little room for additional therapy demands such as swallowing and feeding; however, the incidence of swallowing and feeding disorders in children with developmental disorders has been determined to be between 33% to 80%. These children are in our schools and have swallowing and feeding disorders that prevent them from accessing their curriculum and, as a result, may be preventing them from FAPE. In addition, the incidence of swallowing and feeding disorders in children appears to be occurring more often.

Behavioral feeding disorders present a unique challenge and need to be addressed with a slightly different approach compared to swallowing and feeding disorders that have a safety focus. SLPs, OTs, nurses, BCBA specialists are often employed by school districts and have the knowledge and skills to address these issues. It is within their scope of practice and is clearly within their professional and ethical responsibilities. Behavioral feeding disorders can be managed in school districts by taking a 4 tier approach to prevention, monitoring, direct intervention, and support/referral. By following these steps, students will be safer at school, will be able to participate more fully in their academic program, and will have the opportunity to access to their curriculum throughout the school day. The goals of the behavioral feeding school-based program should be to:

- Identify the underlying causes of the behaviors being observed and to address those issues as they are identified. This includes medical concerns such as gastrointestinal issues, physiological concerns such as oral and pharyngeal dysphagia, oral motor concerns, and sensory processing. In addition, determine where the child is functioning according to feeding developmental motor milestones.
- Decrease mealtime stress for the student, the parents/guardians, and the school staff members.
- Decrease the incidence of problem behaviors at mealtimes in the school setting.
- Increase the student's participation in the school day by ensuring that the child has adequate nutrition and hydration and is able to participate in school meals with peers.
- Advance the student's diet to a more normalized diet for his or her age and developmental level by advancing texture, taste, temperature, and smell.

What Is a Behavioral Feeding Disorder?

Behavioral feeding disorders have been described in the literature as early as 1945/1985 when Kanner first described autism. However, behavioral feeding disorders are not limited to any one group. In the schools there are many students who exhibit a range of feeding disorders. These feeding disorders may be associated with a concurrent swallowing disorder, medical disorder, special education classification, motor, and/or sensory disorder. The range is expansive and therefore a challenge for school districts to determine their role. In addition, it is a very emotional and difficult disorder for families to address. This chapter offers a pragmatic approach to addressing behavioral feeding concerns for school districts that are facing this issue as well as some guidelines for helping families.

According to Schwartz, Corredor, Fisher-Medina, Cohen, and Rabinowitz (2001) the estimates of incidence of feeding problems in normally developing children range from 25% to 45%, while children with developmental delays are known to be at even greater risk. Behavioral feeding disorders rarely occur completely in isolation. Many of these disorders may have originated in children who have been tube fed, have syndromes such as Down syndrome or have autism (Sharp, Jaquess, Morton, & Herzinger, 2010, Twachtman-Reilly, Amaral, & Zebrowski, 2008). Budd et al. (1992) found that the majority of students with behavioral feeding disorders had a combination of organic (those with some form of physiologic causes) and non-organic (environmental, family dynamics, etc.) causes therefore resulting in the need for a comprehensive evaluation of a student's condition rather than one with only a behavioral focus. In addition to significant feeding issues there are often medical, sensory, motor, and cognitive issues, which must be addressed. According to Jenny McGlothlin, MS, CCC/SLP (Newitt, 2013), who runs a feeding program at the University of Texas Dallas-Callier Center for Communication Disorders: "Parents must learn that children's refusal to eat is a form of communication, they are giving us a window into what is wrong with them." It is the responsibility of the professionals who address feeding and the parents to determine the causes of the refusal as well as other behavioral concerns regarding feeding.

School districts have the responsibility to ensure that students have access to their curriculum. Addressing overall behavior disorders in the schools is a large part of every district's special education program. For some children the behavior that will need to be addressed for that child to have FAPE is feeding. Districts need to work closely with families and physicians when addressing behavioral feeding disorders.

Definition of Behavioral Feeding Disorders

A behavioral feeding disorder, for this purpose, is when a child has a response to foods, liquids, and/or mealtimes that interferes with his or her ability to function in normal, daily living activities both at home and in the school setting. A behavioral feeding disorder may manifest itself in children who have an aversion to food and to mealtimes. A child with a behavioral feeding disorder may have a special education classification such as other health impaired, developmental disabilities, or autism, or may be a student who has had many medical issues in infancy, which resulted in an interruption in normal eating development. It is important for the district team to work closely with parents and physicians to investigate the underlying causes of the behaviors.

Signs and Symptoms of Behavioral Feeding Disorders

It is easy to recognize the behaviors related to behavioral feeding disorders. The reported behaviors are usually obvious and can be challenging for the parents/guardians and teachers. These students may exhibit a range of behaviors that result in a limited variety of foods, textures, tastes, and colors. Typically a student is referred for behavioral feeding by either a concerned teacher or parent/guardian. In many cases it is the classroom staff and the district swallowing and feeding team that helps parents to realize that the child's feeding is something that needs to be addressed and that can be helped.

Reports From Parents/Guardians

Parents/guardians may tell school staff that the child prefers to eat only one or two specific foods or food types. They may tell the teacher or the school team evaluator that their child does not enjoy mealtimes and will do things to avoid eating. Some examples of parent reports are:

> " . . . only eats peanut butter, plain bread, yogurt and applesauce. He does not enjoy mealtimes, but he tolerates it."

. . . another parent reported: " . . . her son only eats chicken nuggets, French fries, hash browns, dry cereal and crackers. Everything he eats is crispy and dry."

. . . and another parent remarked: "that her son only eats yogurt, oatmeal, apples, Chester Cheetoes and chicken nuggets. . . . he ate a lot more foods a year ago."

These are typical reports from parent interviews during Child Search evaluations.

Reports From Classroom Teacher/School Team Member

Classroom teachers and their paraprofessionals or classroom assistants are often the first in the schools to notice that a student has a feeding disorder. In many cases they are with the students more than anyone else and become familiar with all of their unique characteristics. There are times when the behaviors that the teachers see in the classroom or school cafeteria are more significant than those reported by the parents/guardians. The expectations and demands of the classroom setting are very different than that of the home. In the school setting students are required to follow routines and schedules. In the home, children may be able to behave or choose what they do more freely than in the school setting. This sometimes results in an escalation of the student's feeding behaviors at school.

Teachers often report the following behaviors: feeding aversion, feeding jags (student only eats one food or one type of food), food refusal, gagging, vomiting, throwing food or utensils, running from food, aggression when presented with food, and overstuffing. Some students may continue to be bottle dependent and/or remain on "baby food" beyond the time it is developmentally appropriate or nutritionally recommended. In some cases they may only eat certain food types and may refuse proteins, vegetables, and other healthy food. The results of these behaviors on the education process and the student's health can be significant. The behavioral feeding disorder will vary in degree, symptoms, and its effect on education. There are instances where the behaviors affect a student's health, resulting in failure to thrive, lethargy, lack of adequate growth, and poor overall health. In other cases, the behaviors may simply be a nuisance. For example, some students will only eat one brand of chips or one brand of chicken nuggets. If they are given these particular foods then they eat and often their weight and health appear to be adequate.

How Much Can a School District Do?

Each district will need to evaluate their resources and determine the level of intervention that they are able to provide. In some districts this may involve contracting out services or referring children to outside agencies. In many districts, they will be able to utilize the trained professionals who are already employed to establish a program to address these needs. School districts are limited to providing services to ensure that students are able to access their curriculum within the school setting and school day. In addition, the district can serve as a support to the home and medical programs that the student receives outside of the school setting and school day.

Identification and Intervention of Behavioral Feeding Disorders: A Complex Process

There are five areas that should be considered when presented with a child that has behavioral feeding concerns in a school system. It is essential that the school team work together to identify the underlying conditions that may be affecting the student's ability to eat and drink. The areas that should be considered are: developmental delays or disorders in feeding, dysphagia, medical issues and concerns, oral sensorimotor concerns, and learned behavioral feeding concerns. Each area must be evaluated to determine the specific issues and concerns each child is experiencing. It is likely that children will have more than one of these concerns, which are contributing to their behaviors during mealtimes. It is essential that a team look at each area to determine the cause of the student's behaviors and to plan an effective treatment regimen (Arts-Rodas & Benoit, 1998).

Working as a Team

The process of identifying and treating children with swallowing and feeding disorders is always a team effort. The team for children with behavioral issues in the school setting includes the SLP, OT, nurse, classroom teacher, paraprofessional/classroom assistant, parent/guardian, and school administrator, and may also include a behavior specialist, BCBA, whenever possible. In addition, the team may need to work with the student's physician, a dietician, a psychologist, and in some cases a feeding disorders clinic. As in the identification and treatment of dysphagia, each team member has a role to play when addressing a behavioral feeding concern.

The team member that serves as the student's case manager will depend on the type of feeding disorder and the areas that are most significant for each child. In all cases it is essential that the team members work together, collaborate, and have a system for communication.

Initiating the Evaluation Process

The first step with any child who is exhibiting swallowing and feeding concerns is for the child to be referred to the Swallowing and Feeding Team within the school district. The Swallowing and Feeding Team Referral Form (see Appendix A) should be completed by the classroom teacher, SLP, OT, or school nurse and turned in to the district administrator. The referral form indicates that the student is having behaviors that are interfering with the child's mealtimes at school. This sets into motion the process for identifying the student's concerns in a systematic, organized manner.

Once the referral has been initiated and a case manager assigned, the case manager calls the parents/guardians to set up a time to interview them regarding their child's swallowing and feeding concerns. The Parent/Guardian Interview Form (see Appendix D) can be used to gather information from the parents/guardian that is essential when evaluating the student's physiological, sensorimotor, medical, and behavioral concerns.

Evaluating the Student's Level of Development in Feeding Skills

The SLP and/or OT evaluate the student's oral motor skills during mealtimes to determine if the student is functioning within the developmental norms for his or her chronological age. The Parent Interview form will be helpful in determining where the student is currently functioning developmentally. The parents/ guardians provide information on the kinds of foods and textures the child eats. In addition, there are questions that pertain to independence when eating, frequency and duration of meals, positioning during feeding, and the utensils the child uses during meals. This information helps the therapists to determine if the child's feeding skills are within normal limits for the child's age.

According to Arvedson (2008) children who have not experienced typical development of oral feeding in the first year of life often require additional time to accept textured food and to make developmentally appropriate gains. Lack of appropriate and successful practice may also result in the loss of previously acquired oral motor skills and/or failure to acquire more advanced skills (Manno, Fox, Eicher, & Kerwin, 2005). Children who are 3 to 5 years old and eating puree may lack the oral motor skills to chew and form a bolus or they may have, as a result of medical issues in infancy, failed to progress beyond the puree stage and be developmentally delayed in their feeding skills. It is important for the school swallowing and feeding team to consider the student's development in relation to milestones relevant to normal feeding. Table 6–1 offers a reference of developmental milestones for feeding that is helpful in identifying children who are delayed in this area. Awareness of where the child is functioning on the developmental chart gives the team information on the student's skills in relation to normal peers and highlights the sequence of development for feeding. It is essential that swallowing and feeding team members are famil-

Table 6–1. Milestones Relevant to Normal Feeding

Age (months)	Progression of Liquid and Food	Oral-Motor Skills	Motor Skills
Birth to 4	• Liquid	• Suckle on nipple	• Head control develops
4 to 6	• Purees	• Suckle off spoon • Progress from suckle to suck	• Sitting balance • Hands to midline • Hand-to-mouth play
6 to 9	• Purees • Soft chewables	• Cup drinking with assistance • Vertical munching • Limited lateral tongue movements	• Reach, pincer grasp • Assists with spoon • Finger feeding begins
9 to 12	• Ground • Lumpy purees	• Increased independent cup drinking	• Refines pincer grasp • Finger feeding • Grasps spoon with whole hand
12 to 18	• All textures	• Lateral tongue action • Diagonal chew • Straw drinking	• Independent feeding increases • Scoops food, brings to mouth
18 to 24	• More chewable food	• Rotary chewing • Decrease in food intake by 24 months	• Increased control of utensils
24+	• Tougher solids	• Increase in mature chewing for tougher solids	• Total self-feeding • Increased use of fork • Cup drinking, open cup, and no spilling

Source: Reprinted from *Clinical Practice Guideline, Report of the Recommendations, Motor Disorders, Assessment and Intervention for Young Children (Ages 0–3 Years),* 2006, with permission of the New York State Department of Health. Adapted from Arvedson, 1996.

iar with normal developmental milestones for feeding because expectations for chewing are based on these milestones (New York State Department of Health, 2006).

Medical Issues Associated With Swallowing and Feeding Disorders

There are many medical concerns, outside of dysphagia, that could be contributing to a child's refusal to eat. The school nurse is instrumental in working with the team to determine if the child is having medical issues. The first step in the process of ruling out medical conditions is for the Parent/Guardian Interview Form (see Appendix D) to be completed and discussed with the parent/guardian. The speech pathologist, occupational therapist, or school nurse may conduct this interview. It is recommended that the interview take place face to face, if possible. Relevant information that is gathered from this interview includes the following: a list of the physicians who are currently treating the student; student's history of allergies, bowel habits, medical tests such as MBSS/VFSS and upper GI; failure to thrive; feeding tube; hospitalizations; and dental; list of medications the student currently takes; and current feeding practices. This interview gives the nurse information that guides the evaluation of the child's current medical condition as it relates to feeding. Some factors that may contribute to a behavioral feeding disorder are: GERD, slow or delayed gastric emptying, contraindications of medicines, mouth ulcers, constipation, frequent vomiting, no physical sensation of hunger or thirst, physical discomfort when eating or drinking, small window of time until satiation, hypersensitive gag reflex, allergies, and dental problems. Whenever it appears that the child is in physical discomfort when eating or drinking, it is recommended that a physician evaluate and treat the child to further rule out any potential medical issues.

Addressing Medical Issues

If the nurse determines that there are medical issues, which could be contributing or are contributing to a student's feeding behaviors then it will be necessary for her or him to work closely with the student's parents/guardians. The school nurse discusses with the parents/guardians concerns that have come up during the evaluation of the student's feeding. These concerns may result in the need for follow-up by a physician, dentist, psychologist, or other professional. In order for the school district team to talk with the student's medical professional, it is necessary to have a release of information form signed by the parents/guardians. This form, when signed, allows the nurse or other designated school system professionals to call and discuss their concerns with the child's medical team. In order for this to occur the school team must have a positive relationship with the parents/guardians that is based on trust and mutual interest in the child's well-being. In cases where the nurse has concerns that medical issues may be contributing to the student's feeding disorders the following actions should be taken:

- Determine the type of medial referral that may be indicated.
- Facilitate communication by recommending that parents/ guardians discuss the issues with the child's physician, dentist, pharmacist, dietician, and so forth.
- Monitor the student's weight by completing a growth profile, baseline weight, and a subsequent weekly nurse's evaluation and weight measure.
- Look at the student's medications to determine if side effects or the combination of medicines could be affecting the student's appetite or ability to enjoy food. Some medications affect a student's appetite such as: steroids, atypical antipsychotics, mood stabilizers, tricyclic antidepressants, anticonvulsants, and stimulants (Bandini et al., 2011). Communication with the student's parents/guardians and physicians is indicated for children on these medications who are exhibiting some behavioral feeding characteristics.

Any suspected medical conditions should be addressed immediately; however, the behavioral evaluation may continue in order to address learned behaviors that have occurred as the result of the initial medical concerns. In some cases, the behaviors interfere so significantly that they will need to be addressed at school while medical treatment is occurring. It should be noted that many behaviors associated with a feeding disorder might be attributed to medical issues, especially gastrointestinal disorders such as GERD. Studies by Schwartz et al. (2001) revealed gastroesophageal reflux (GER) with or without aspiration in 44 of 79 patients, 56% of students studied with behavioral feeding signs and symptoms. Most of these were able to be addressed with medical treatment such as GER therapy or fundoplicaton.

Identifying Accompanying Dysphagia Concerns

The school district that has an interdisciplinary swallowing and feeding team in place and has developed a system-wide team procedure will follow their procedure to identify any dysphagia issues. Once the referral, parent/guardian interview, and nurse's evaluation are completed, the team conducts the Interdisciplinary Observation (see Appendix E) to determine other swallowing and feeding concerns. The team observes the student eating a typical meal; including liquids and foods that are part of his typical diet. Many students will have oral, pharyngeal, and/or esophageal dysphagia in addition to other feeding issues and concerns. These swallowing safety issues must always be considered and addressed when present in a student with feeding behaviors. The safety issues always take precedence over behavioral or sensory concerns. Refer to Chapter 3 in this book to follow the procedure for identifying dysphagia. Included in that procedure are also the steps required for identification of a behavioral feeding disorder.

Identifying Sensory Issues Which Contribute to Behaviors During Mealtimes

Many behavioral feeding disorders will be rooted in accompanying oral sensorimotor issues. In many cases it will be necessary to address both the sensorimotor and the behavioral issues at the same time. It is necessary to begin figuring out the issues surrounding the student's behaviors by evaluating the student's sensory status. Though behavioral issues may develop secondary to sensorimotor problems in the mouth, we need to consider the child's refusal as an adaptive, communicative response to a negative experience, rather than as the primary disability to be addressed (Overland, 2011). Overland stresses the importance of both sensory and motor skill assessment and treatment. Assessment and treatment of the underlying sensorimotor issues should, in many cases, precede behavioral interventions.

Typically and whenever possible an SLP or OT should conduct a sensorimotor screening (see Appendix E). One of the first steps in determining if there are sensory issues will be to complete the Sensory Questionnaire and Observation Form, which is part of the Interdisciplinary Observation discussed in Chapter 3. A sensory screening will look at food texture, temperature, and taste. In addition, hyposensitivity versus hypersensitivity should also be considered.

Signs of a Sensory Disorder

Sensory disorders associated with feeding typically manifest themselves in one or more of 3 areas: taste, texture, and temperature.

Taste—children only eat one type of food such as salty, sweet, sour, bland.

Texture—children avoid eating foods that have any texture at all or are limited to eating only one texture, such as puree foods, crunchy foods, or liquids. When presented with a different food texture they have a negative reaction.

Temperature—some children will be hypersensitive to foods of certain temperatures such as foods that are warm (oatmeal) or cold (ice cream) and only eat foods at room temperature.

Any of these sensory conditions may result in the reporting of behaviors such as: refusing foods, tantrums, and screaming. It takes a trained specialist to determine if there is a sensory component to the student's behavior. The OT is trained to determine if the sensory issues that are being observed during mealtimes also occur in other sensory situations such as sensitivity to certain fabrics or colors of clothing.

Oral Hypersensitivity. Children with oral and/or facial hypersensitivity react to being touched or to food being presented in or around the mouth or face. These children will resist brushing their teeth, washing their face, or new food textures. They may not like to be touched in the oral area or even on the rest of their body, and they often do not want to use utensils for eating. Some of these children gag easily when presented with new food textures or foods that they are sensitive to.

Oral Hyposensitivity. Child with low sensitivity may also have feeding issues. These children often prefer foods with strong tastes such as spicy, salty, and sour. They overstuff because of their inability to feel the amount of food inside their mouth. They frequently pocket their food, which could be interpreted as food refusal but may actually be a result of their low sensitivity. They are at risk for choking because they frequently swallow their food without adequately chewing. These children often have food on their faces after they eat and may be messy eaters.

Identifying Developmental Motor Delays Which Contribute to Behaviors During Mealtimes

Children develop feeding skills such as sucking, munching, and rotary chew, within a set of developmental norms. According to Sheppard (2008) developmental milestones for eating are defined by transitions between types of foods (liquids to soft, etc.), type of utensils (bottles to spoons), and independence (holding bottle, feeding with fingers, etc.). The primary milestones are generally considered to be nippling, eating from a spoon, drinking from a cup, sipping from a straw, biting, chewing, and self-feeding. When this developmental process is interrupted or does not occur for any variety of reasons, then a child may be asked to handle foods that he or she is not motorically or developmentally able to do. This can result in negative responses to eating, which then develops into some of the behaviors that are observed later when the student enters school. It is important to take into consideration where the child is functioning in the developmental stages of chewing, swallowing, drinking, and so forth. Any breakdown in oral sensory-motor development can result in gagging, choking, vomiting, and subsequent food refusal (Twachtmen-Reilly, Amaral, & Zebrowski, 2008). These developmental delays may also be evident in speech and fine and gross motor skills. Responding to the delay by providing foods and textures that are appropriate for the child's developmental level helps to eliminate some of the problem behaviors.

Signs of a Developmental Oral Motor Delay and/or Oral Motor Disorder

Children who are delayed in achieving the developmental milestones for eating typically remain at an earlier eating stage. For example, they may continue to only be able to tolerate puree foods, such as Stage 1 baby foods, and have difficulty manipulating foods with textures or have trouble keeping some foods in their mouths. They may continue to depend on bottle-feeding and be resistant to or unable to maneuver spoon-feeding. Chewing skills may resemble munching as opposed to the rotary chewing that develops later. With all developmental norms there is some variability as to when children move through the stages; however, if a child remains at one level too long the pattern may be established and more difficult to address.

Some children have oral motor disorders, which affect their ability to chew and swallow within normal limits. These children often limit the textures and foods that they eat because of difficulty adequately chewing and forming a cohesive bolus. When determining if a child has an oral motor disorder, the SLP or OT will want to observe a child's facial features noting symmetry and asymmetry of the lips and jaw, the palate height and shape, tongue position in the oral cavity, and tongue movement patterns (Arvedson, 2008). A thorough oral mechanism examination should be performed if a therapist suspects an oral motor disorder.

Discriminating Between Disorders That Are Primarily Oral Sensory From Those That Are Primarily Oral Motor

It is necessary when evaluating students to determine if what you are looking at is the result of a sensorimotor disorder or primarily an oral motor disorder. They often can appear to be the same. The child with an oral motor disorder will consistently have difficulty with foods regardless of their taste, texture, and temperature. Reactions to foods often occur once the food is in the oral cavity, whereas with sensorimotor children the reaction is often at the presence of the food. According to Overland (2011), children with muscle-based issues that affect feeding often use compensatory movements such as wide jaw excursions, tongue protrusion, and jaw/lover lip protrusions. The child with an oral motor disorder will consistently have difficulty with foods and textures as compared to the sensory student whose difficulty appears to be more selective and less consistent.

Determining if the Behaviors Are Consistent With Other Behavioral Issues at School and at Home

The final task in diagnosing a behavioral feeding disorder in the schools is to look at the child's total behavior profile. This will require an observation by a trained specialist in behavior to determine if the behaviors that are seen at mealtimes also occur throughout the day in other situations. At this point, someone will need to look at the behaviors that are occurring and determine if they are being reinforced by the reactions they are receiving and if those behaviors are consistent to the child's overall behavior issues. The behavior specialists (or other trained personnel) should ask the following questions when determining the presence and extent of a student's feeding behaviors:

- Are the behaviors that they are observing the result of the student's desire or need to escape or avoid a situation?
- Are the behaviors that they are observing the result of the student's need for attention? It can be positive or negative attention.
- Is the purpose of the behaviors they are observing for the student to obtain a tangible object such as a toy, money, or activity?
- Does the student use these same behaviors throughout the day for activities other than mealtimes or feeding?

Some students have behaviors that only occur during mealtimes or when food is presented. Some of the more common behaviors unique to feeding behaviors that are reported are:

pushing food away, throwing food, turning away, crying, saying "No!" refusing to open mouth, expelling foods from mouth, and gagging and/or vomiting.

The treatment of the disorder depends on the extent of the behaviors in the course of the student's day as well as the degree and severity of them. Box 6–1 summarizes the procedure for diagnosing behavioral feeding disorders in the schools.

Box 6–1. Summary of Procedures for Diagnosing Behavioral Feeding Disorders in the Schools

Areas Addressed in the Evaluation Process

- Stages of development in feeding
- Physiological issues and concerns (dysphagia)
- Medical issues and concerns
- Oral motor and sensorimotor skills
- Behavioral concerns related to foods, feeding, and mealtimes

Procedure for Identifying and Treating Behavioral Feeding Disorders in the School Setting

- Initial referral by school staff and/or parents/guardians
- Parent/guardian interview and history
- Evaluation of student's level of development in feeding skills based on his or her age.
  - ○ Types of foods tolerated
  - ○ Types of utensils currently using
  - ○ Level of independence when eating
- Evaluation of swallowing and feeding skills:
  - ○ Clinical evaluation for **dysphagia**, including observation of liquids and foods presented
  - ○ Clinical observation of **sensorimotor skills** and reactions during mealtimes
  - ○ Clinical observation of **behaviors** when foods are presented
- Nursing evaluation of student's medical status including current conditions, medications, dental care, and allergies.

- Follow up on **medical conditions**:
  - Communication with parents/guardians regarding student's medical concerns related to feeding
  - Medical referral when indicated including: gastroenterologist, dentist, neurologist, and/or psychologist or psychiatrist
  - Monitor student's weight and height, completing a growth profile and weekly nurse's evaluations and weight measures.
  - Investigate student's medications and the effect they may have on the student's appetite or ability to enjoy food.
- Plan for addressing issues and concerns is written:
  - Swallowing and feeding plan
  - Functional behavioral analysis of feeding skills
  - Behavior intervention plan for feeding
- Swallowing and feeding plan including behavior plan is implemented.

A Four-Tier Hierarchy Model for Classifying and Treating Behavioral Feeding

There are many benefits to seeing children within a school system. Children are in school all day, every day, and for many years. School personnel have the opportunity to work with them over long periods of time. Districts see children of all ages and severity, which requires many levels of service to meet their needs. A four-tier hierarchy model is suggested to address the various levels of intervention that school districts encounter (Table 6–2).

Tier 1: Proactive/Prevention of Feeding Disorders

Whether we are looking at language disorders, academic issues, or feeding, the ideal situation is to be proactive and prevent a problem from occurring. IDEA requires that school districts screen and evaluate children starting at 3 years old. School districts can

Table 6–2. Hierarchy of Levels of Feeding Concern

Tier 4: Disordered

Behaviors are severe, consistent and often have the potential of affecting the student's health. They are at a great risk of being failure to thrive and are often below 5th percentile in weight. Health risks are present and district works with family and physician supporting feeding program.

Tier 3: Problem Feeders

Behaviors interfere with the child getting a well-balanced meal at school and/or sufficient nutrition, as well as interfering with academic and social programs at school. Direct intervention by the swallowing and feeding team and behavior specialist to progress diet and nutrition at school.

Tier 2: Picky Eaters

Eats foods from the four major food groups, will touch or taste new foods and tolerate new food on their plate. Typically eat at least one food from most food textures. Limit the amounts and variety of food that they eat. Consultation services and packet of information given to parents of students who report picky eating characteristics during evaluation process.

Tier 1: Proactive—Family Centered

Students are typical eaters. General nutrition information distributed to parents/guardians of students in Child Find.

Source: Adapted from St. Tammany Parish Schools Swallowing and Feeding Team, Covington, Louisiana.

serve as an information source for parents regarding feeding and nutrition. At the Tier 1 level, it is recommended that the parents/ guardians of all children who are screened for speech/language and/or learning disorders are given public service information on good nutrition and mealtime practice. At this level, parents are given suggestions for getting children to eat a variety of foods. This "good parenting" type of information can be presented at the screening level, during the intake interview, or as part of the packet of information that is given to a parent or guardian as they leave. The goal is to get families talking about good nutrition with children. This is a great time to discuss with parents the importance of good nutrition on development and learning and to share with them the following:

- Nutritional information provided by the United States Department of Agriculture Food and Nutrition Service. The website, http://www.choosemyplate.gov, provides printable pamphlets and brochures that school districts can share with families.
- Additional take home information is available online through http://www.fns.usda.gov. There are games and activities for exploring healthy choices, learning about fruits and vegetables and how they grow, selecting balanced meals, and more. They offer games, such as videos and activities for children and their families to discover nutrition at home in a relaxed, fun way!

Tier 2: Picky Eaters

The next level of student is what is referred to as "picky eaters." This group of students often will eat foods from each of the four major food groups, will touch or taste new foods, and will tolerate new foods on their plate. Typically they eat at least one food from most food textures; however, while these students basically have a balanced diet, they limit the amounts of food that they eat and have a limited variety of foods in their diets.

According to the Children's Health Network (http://www .childrenshealthnetwork.org) children are most typically picky eaters during the toddler and preschool years. Characteristics of picky eaters are: complaining and whining; refusing certain foods, especially meats and vegetables; pushing foods around the plate; and hiding foods or giving them to the pet. In spite of these behaviors, these children typically consume adequate calories and nutrition for normal growth. According to the Mayo Clinic (http://www.mayoclinic.org) how a parent reacts to a child's picky eating can actually promote "picky eating." For example, preparing a separate meal for the child, after the child has rejected the family meal may actually encourage picky eating in a young child.

In a national random sample of 3,022 infants and toddlers, Carruth, Ziegler, Gordon, and Barr (2004) found that the percentage of children identified by their caregivers as picky eaters was 50% by age 24 months. These reported observations included all ages, ethnicities, and household incomes. According to their caregivers, although picky eating is really prevalent among typically developing children; this behavior may put these children at a higher risk for developing into a problem feeder. In the school system we can serve as an information source to parents/guardians who report eating issues with their toddler or preschooler. As a Tier 2 level intervention, the team evaluating preschool students will provide consultation services or will recommend that the school team provide consultative services to parents/guardians who report a concern with their child's picky eating. Like Tier 1, this is a proactive approach to preventing more serious feeding issues, but it is a more direct intervention. A school district can prepare a packet of information to give to parents during a one-time consultation service. This packet of information may include the following:

- Information on dealing with a picky eater
- List of websites that tell parents/guardians tips for dealing with picky eaters.
- Brochure or list of books that present stories for and about young children who are picky eaters. (For an example see: http://www.perrotlibrary.org/book_brochures/picky_eaters_brochure.pdf)
- Provide for parents a book such as Burger Boy (Durant, 2005) or Tales for Very Picky Eaters (Schneider, 2011) that is about children who are picky eaters. This information

is given to families who report behaviors that are characteristic of picky eaters during the evaluation.
- SLPs demonstrate to parents/guardians reading the story to their preschooler in a way that encourages positive food attitudes.

After the one-time consultation service is provided to the parents/guardians, the parents/guardians are encouraged to contact the swallowing and feeding team if the child's feeding behaviors get worse. This opens the line of communication with the family.

Tier 3: Problem Feeders

Problem feeders may be the group that the swallowing and feeding team comes in contact with most frequently. These students have developed behaviors that interfere with their academic and social program at school. The behaviors reported with problem feeders interfere with the child getting a well-balanced meal at school and/or sufficient nutrition. Medical issues and dysphagia have been addressed and are managed as soon as they are identified. There are many different types of behaviors that will be observed or reported. Some of the more common behaviors are that the student:

- Cries or acts out when presented with new food
- Refuses entire categories of food textures
- Avoids one or more food groups
- Exhibits unusual aversions
- Demonstrates tactile and oral defensiveness
- Runs or tries to escape from the food or from eating (Weaver, 2008)

At this point, the student's behavior has been learned to the degree that, without intervention, the behaviors could worsen and the student's health could be compromised. Sensory and motor issues have been identified and are part of the intervention plan. The intervention process includes several members of the swallowing and feeding team working collaboratively to decrease the behaviors, address the sensory and motor issues, manage nutrition, and progress the student's diet at school.

Problem feeders will need direct therapy to address desensitizing them to new textures, tastes, smells, and/or temperatures, and gradually adding to their tolerance for a variety of foods. The speech-language pathologist, the occupational therapist, the behavior specialist, the classroom teacher, and/or the paraprofessionals in the classroom are all responsible to some degree in providing this the intervention. The student will experience more success if the parents/guardians are trained to follow up on feeding strategies at home.

Direct Intervention Based on Evaluation Results

The evaluation process described previously should provide the school team with the information they need to develop an intervention program at school. Once the medical issues are addressed or have been referred to a physician, the school swallowing and feeding team makes decisions on interventions to address other areas of concern. If the student has dysphagia issues, then a swallowing and feeding plan has been established to ensure safe feeding at school, since this is done immediately after identifying oral and/or pharyngeal concerns. This plan takes into consideration the information from the student's evaluation on the oral and pharyngeal phases of the swallow. Any behavior interventions will have to adhere to the restrictions in the dysphagia plan. Esophageal issues and concerns should have already been addressed through the medical portion of the evaluation.

Prior to beginning a feeding intervention, a few guidelines are recommended. These guidelines for the most part apply to all children with behavioral feeding concerns:

- Mealtimes and food experience in general should be pleasant and stress free.
- The goals should focus on adequate nutrition and hydration for health and growth.
- The mealtime environment for the child with behavioral feeding issues may need to be quiet and distraction free, at least initially.

Student Profile George: Behavioral Feeding Disorder

George was born premature and at one year old was diagnosed with hydrocephalus and a shunt was surgically inserted. He came to the school district as a 3-year-old weighing 20 pounds. His parents packed his lunch, which consisted of Stage 1 baby food, mostly sweet fruits and deserts. The school team met with the parents and presented a plan for expanding his diet. At that point the parents only gave him the foods he liked and were not interested in expanding his diet. Reluctantly they gave the school team permission to try different foods during the school day. The school team made efforts that year to introduce different foods but George only attended school 3 half days a week, parent "buy in" was weak, and progress was minimal.

The following school year he was full time at school and the family was more concerned and receptive to feeding therapy. The swallowing and feeding team worked closely with his mother to expand his diet to include more nutritious choices and to increase the amount of food he ate at school. They began by doing an activity with the mom where she identified the foods that he was currently eating into one of two categories: snack type foods or meal type foods. George only had a couple of items on the meal type foods. This was an awakening for the mom who was then ready to work with the team.

The SLP began by having food available during language therapy to help desensitize him to new foods. Initially it was on the table, but eventually he touched it, licked it, and tasted it. The team then started pureeing foods similar to what he was already eating (e.g., pureed fresh peaches). He continued to throw tantrums when presented with different foods. At the same time the school observed that George used tantrums to escape whatever he was asked to do that he did not want to do. The behavioral specialist was called in and a behavior plan was written that addressed his behaviors throughout the day, including feeding. George progressed slowly to include different, more nutritious foods and textures into his diet. The behavior plan was effective and George is now performing better across his curriculum.

Many children will have some degree of oral sensorimotor delays as well as developmental delays. For these children the interventions are often similar. The following techniques and procedures can be used for children who are not progressing through textures, tastes, and temperatures and who have limited food variety.

- Establish a mealtime routine both at school and at home. When possible, have the child eat with his or her family and peers.
- Work closely with the parents/guardians for carryover of feeding into the home and school setting.
- Begin with foods that are similar to the ones the child is already eating successfully.
- Introduce the nonpreferred food before giving the student the food that the child is already successfully eating or present the preferred and nonpreferred foods at the same time.
- Follow the developmental sequence when moving through different stages for food textures, use of utensils, and feeding independence.
- Only introduce one taste, texture, temperature, or color food at a time
- Allow the student to experience the food without actually putting it in his or her mouth, such as touching it, allowing it on the table, and licking it.
- If the child is tube fed, work on eating before he or she receives the tube feeding.
- Be patient, this process will go very slowly

Tier 4: Disordered Feeder

At the top of the hierarchy of levels of feeding disorders are the students referred to as disordered feeders. These students have behaviors that are severe, consistent, and often are affecting the student's health. In the disordered feeder the refusal behaviors are more severe than in problem feeders and need more intense intervention. In these cases the school district is typically a small part of the bigger picture of health and nutrition. These children are at a great risk of being failure to thrive and are often below the 5th percentile in weight. The severity of their feeding disorder can affect the student's participation in the educational setting in a number of ways:

- Student may be so disruptive during any situation where food is presented (i.e., breakfast, snack, lunch, etc.) that he or she is not able to participate and socialize with their peers during meals.
- Student may lack adequate nutrition and/or hydration and not have the stamina to participate in his or her academic program.
- Student's poor nutrition may prevent him or her from attending school.
- Student's poor nutrition may result in minimal growth and development.

These are serious issues, which need the attention of the student's family and physicians as well as the school team's support. In some cases, the student's behaviors may be the result of anxiety that requires the services of a medical professional to address food anxieties. The school system should work closely with the medical professionals addressing these issues as well as with the parents/guardians.

The school-based team's interventions are similar to the problem feeder, working to expand the student's diet and nutrition and decrease the behaviors that interfere with successful mealtimes. This student, in some cases, has additional disruptive behaviors that may result in the need for the behavioral specialist or BCBA to serve as the swallowing and feeding case manager. There are different approaches to addressing the severe feeding behaviors of the disordered feeder, but in all approaches the role of the school district is limited to the affect the disorder has on the student's educational program.

Behavior Modification (Applied Behavioral Analysis) Approach

For children whose feeding disorders are so severe that they put their health and well-being at risk, there are special feeding clinics and feeding therapy specialists in most communities. Many feeding clinics and feeding programs are associated with university programs or hospitals and often use the principles of applied behavioral analysis to systematically train the child to eat. There are also independent, private facilities, and therapists who also work on severe feeding disorders using ABA principles. This approach is based on the principles of behavior modification and follows the structure of the Behavior Intervention Plan that is developed in school systems to address student's behavior issues. Instructional techniques such as shaping, modeling, prompting and prompt fading, and size fading are used to extinguish the maladaptive eating behaviors and establish more appropriate behaviors.

Student Profile: Intense Feeding Clinic

Paul was born with a diaphragmatic hernia that caused his left lung to be underdeveloped. As a result of his early illness and his difficulty digesting food, a PEG tube was inserted around 2 years old for "failure to thrive." He entered the school district as a 3-year-old who relied completely on tube feeding for all nutrition and hydration. When Paul was four, the physician wanted to wean him from the tube (he was not at risk for aspiration). He had not been getting any food or drink orally for over a year and had an extreme reaction to oral feeding. The OT and SLP at his school worked directly on desensitizing him to tastes and textures but he did not respond to any of the interventions. The parents became very concerned and had the means to take him to an intensive, private feeding clinic. This clinic addressed his feeding issues intensively using ABA principles and Paul was weaned from the tube within a month. When he returned to the school district, the school team was responsible for continuing the very strict feeding protocol that was established at the clinic. The clinic staff periodically saw the student and the program from the clinic continued to work toward more normalized eating. The school district followed the recommended program and Paul, currently in 5th grade, eats normal cafeteria meals at school. Paul did not enjoy eating during this process and still does not appear to enjoy food; however, he is healthy and able to eat with his peers at school.

Even with the most severe cases, it is important that food be presented in a pleasurable setting if possible. A combination of approaches that utilize the knowledge and skills of speech-language pathologists and occupational therapists working along with behavioral specialists, psychologists, and parents/guardians provides the best opportunity for students to successfully transition to more normalized mealtimes.

Summary of School Behavioral Feeding Services

This chapter has provided a system for identifying behavioral feeding disorders and addressing them in the school setting. It is important to recognize that the school system is only one facet in a multifaceted approach to identifying and treating this disorder. It is essential that the district work closely with the parents/guardians and physicians treating the student to ensure that the child's program is consistent throughout and that all areas are addressed. There are five areas that must be assessed in order to determine why the student is exhibiting the problem behaviors. These areas are: developmental motor delays or disorders related to feeding, dysphagia concerns, medical issues and concerns, oral sensorimotor concerns, and learned behavioral feeding concerns. Each area must be evaluated and addressed in order to ensure that the cause of the behaviors has been identified and can then be treated in the most effective and efficient manner possible.

A school system can use a four-tier approach to treat behavioral feeding disorders. The first two tiers use a proactive approach to prevent mild eating preferences from progressing into feeding problems. The third tier addresses problem feeders and will require direct therapeutic intervention by the school team. The final tier is comprised of the smallest number of students and usually requires a team management that includes the school team as a support. Regardless of the level of intervention or of the severity of the feeding concerns, the school district can play a role in helping students to receive adequate nutrition and hydration while at school.

References

Arts-Rodas, D., & Benoit, D. (1998). Feeding problems in infancy and early childhood: Identification and management. *Paediatrics and Child Health, 3*(1), 21–27.

Arvedson, J. (2008). Assessment of pediatric dysphagia and feeding disorders: Clinical and instrumental approaches. *Developmental Disabilities Research Reviews, 14,* 118–127.

Bandini, L., Anderson, S., Curtin, C., Cermak, S., Evans, E., Scampini, R., . . . Must, A. (2011). Food selectivity in children with autism spectrum disorders and typically developing children. *Journal of Pediatrics, 157*(2), 259–264.

Budd, K. S., McGraw, T. E., Farbisz, R., Murphy, T. B., Hawkins, D., . . . Werle, M. (1992). Psychosocial concomitants of children's feeding disorders. *Journal of Pediatric Psychology, 17,* 81–94.

Carruth, B. R., Ziegler, P. J., Gordon, A., & Barr, S. I. (2004). Prevalence of picky eaters among infants and toddlers and their caregivers' decisions about offering a new food. *Journal of the American Dietetic Association, 10*(1), S57–S64.

Durant, A. (2005). *Burger boy* (pp. 1–29). New York, NY: Clarion Books.

Kanner, L. (1985). Autistic disturbances of affective contact. In A. M. Donnellan (Ed.), *Classic readings in autism* (pp. 11–50). New York, NY: Teachers College Press. (Reprinted from *Childhood psychosis: Initial studies and new insights* (pp. 1–43), by L. Kanner (Ed.), 1973, Washington, DC: V. H. Winston; original work published in *Nervous Child, 2* (1943), 217–250.)

Manno, C. J., Fox, C., Eicher, P. S., & Kerwin, M. E. (2005). Early oral-motor interventions for pediatric feeding problems: What, when and how. *Journal of Early and Intensive Behavior Intervention, 2*(3), 145–159.

Newitt, V. N. (2013). *Considering the whole child, not just behaviors, is vital to effective feeding therapy.* King of Prussia, PA: ADVANCE Newsmagazines. Retrieved from https://speech-language-pathology-audiology.advanceweb.com/Features/Articles/Feeding-Disorders.aspx

New York State Department of Health. (2006). *Clinical practice guideline: Report of the recommendations. Motor Disorders, Assessment and Intervention for Young Children (Age 0–3 Years).* Publication No. 4962.

Overland, L. (2011). *A sensory-motor approach to feeding.* Retrieved from http://journals.asha.org/perspectives/terms.dtl

Schneider, J. (2011). *Tales for very picky eaters* (pp. 1–47). New York, NY: Clarion Books.

Schwartz, S. M., Corredor, J., Fisher-Medina, J., Cohen, J., & Rabinowitz, S. (2001). Diagnosis and treatment of feeding disorders in children with developmental disabilities, *Pediatrics, 108*(3), 671–676.

Sharp, W. G., Jaquess, D. L., Morton, J. F., & Herzinger, C. V. (2010). Pediatric feeding disorders: A quantitative synthesis of treatment outcomes. *Clinical Child and Family Psychology Review, 13*(4), 348–365.

Sheppard, J. (2008). Using motor learning approaches for treating swallowing and feeding disorders: A review. *Language, Speech, and Hearing Services in Schools, 39*, 227–236.

Twachtman-Reilly, J., Amaral, S. C., & Zebrowski. P. (2008). Addressing feeding disorders in children on the autism spectrum in school-based settings: Physiological and behavioral issues. *Language, Speech, and Hearing Services in Schools, 39*, 261–272. doi:10.1044/0161-1461(2008/025)

Weaver, C. (2008). *Evaluation and management of behavioral-based and sensory-based feeding problems.* American Speech-Language-Hearing Association annual convention, Chicago, IL.

Websites

Children's Health Network:
http://www.childrenshealthnetwork.org

Mayo Clinic: http://www.mayoclinic.org

Perrot Library:
http://www.perrotlibrary.org/book_brochures/picky_eaters_brochure.pdf

Picky Eater Tips:
http://pediasure.com/kid-nutrition/picky-eater-tips

Picky Eater Slide Show:
http://www.webmd.com/parenting/ss/slideshow-picky-eaters

Sensory Processing Disorder:
http://www.sensory-processing-disorder.com

Tips for Preschoolers Who Are Picky Eaters: http://www.pbs.org/parents/special/article-nutrition-picky.html

United States Department of Agriculture, National Agricultural Library: http://fnic.nal.usda.gov/consumers/ages-stages

7

Addressing Nutrition in the School Setting

Emily M. Homer

Introduction

When a person has swallowing and feeding concerns, regardless of the setting, nutrition and hydration must be considered. This chapter addresses the role of a school district in meeting the nutritional needs of students with swallowing and feeding disorders. The goal is to ensure that students with swallowing and feeding issues are receiving adequate nutrition and hydration while attending school.

The National School Lunch Program

In order to understand how students with swallowing and feeding disorders in the school setting receive the nutrition and hydration that they need to be successful at school, it may be helpful to understand the National School Lunch Program. According to its official website, the National School Lunch Program is a federally assisted meal program operating in public schools, nonprofit private schools, and residential child-care institutions.

It provides nutritionally balanced, low-cost or free lunches to children each school day.

History of the National School Lunch Program

A book written in 1904, *Poverty* by Robert Hunter, pointed out that "learning is difficult because hungry stomachs and languid bodies and thin blood are not able to feed the brain. The lack of learning among so many poor children is certainly due, to an important extent, to this cause" (Gunderson, 2014). Reportedly this book had a strong influence upon the U.S. effort to feed hungry, needy children in school. Through the turn of the century and the early 1900s, individual cities and states began providing some meals at no cost to children attending schools. Some of these programs were provided by charitable organizations. The school lunch movement continued to spread with more districts around the country offering some form of nutrition to children at school.

By 1937, 15 states had passed laws specifically authorizing local school boards to operate lunchrooms primarily to poor students either free or at low cost. The program that we are familiar with today was established under the National School Lunch Act, signed by President Harry Truman in 1946. In recent years, based on input from teachers and school administrators, the focus of the school lunch program is nutrition. Teachers and administrators observed that when children ate healthier meals that they were able to concentrate better and learn more. The National School Lunch program now has nutrition guides for parents as well as a new focus on using fresh, made-from-scratch foods as well as seasonal fruits and vegetables. The importance of students eating healthy nutritious meals at school applies to all students including those with swallowing and feeding disorders (U.S. Department of Agriculture, 2014).

National School Lunch Program Nutritional Guidelines

In July 2012, school meal programs began implementing new standards for addressing school nutrition. The proposed rule sought to increase the availability of fruits, vegetables, whole grains, and fat-free and low-fat fluid milk in the school menu; reduce the levels of sodium, saturated fat and trans fat in school meals; and meet the nutrition needs of school children within their calorie requirements. The intent of the proposed rule was to provide nutrient-dense meals (high in nutrients and low in calories) to better meet the dietary needs of school children and protect their health (Department of Agriculture, 2012). More than ever, students have access to healthy nutritious meals during the school day at little or no cost. All federally funded school meal programs must meet the regulations issued by the Federal Register. As a result, school lunch programs are very similar in what they offer students.

School Meal Programs issue monthly menus that identify the meals that will be offered to students throughout the month. Typically, a district will issue one monthly plan and they will repeat it throughout the year with some changes in the days meals are offered and in the fresh seasonal fruits and vegetables that may be available (Table 7–1).

Providing a Nutritious Meal for Students With Swallowing and Feeding Disorders

Cafeteria School Meals: A Team Effort

Many children with swallowing and feeding disorders eat two of their meals at school. Once a swallowing and feeding plan is established, it is essential that the school team, usually the case manager, work closely with the classroom and cafeteria staff. If a child needs an alteration to the school cafeteria meal, it is a federal regulation that the district gets a Prescription of School Meal Modification Form (see Appendix G) completed by the student's physician. This allows the cafeteria to make the changes necessary to address the student's individual needs while at the same time maintaining good nutritional status. The process of providing a modification to a child's meal in the school cafeteria will take a team of school personnel.

Table 7–1. Sample Elementary School Cafeteria Menu K–6

	Monday	Tuesday	Wednesday	Thursday	Friday
Week 1					
Meat	Red Beans, White Beans, Gumbo, or Jambalaya	Tacos, Gordita, (beef or chicken) with Cheese	Catfish, Fish Strips, or Square	Chicken Tenderloin	Hamburger or Sliders, BBQ Chicken or Chicken Patty/Sliders (choice of 2 sand.)
Fruit	Frozen Fruit Sorbet	Fresh Fruit Choice	Fresh or Canned Fruit Choice	Fresh Fruit Choice	Fresh or Canned Fruit Choice
Vegetables	Spinach or Fresh Broccoli Carrot Sticks or Rounds	Green Leaf Lettuce Salsa	Raw Broccoli Mashed Potatoes or Baked Potato— White and/or Sweet	Salad Mixed Vegetables	Green Leaf Lettuce Potato Rounds or Fries
Legumes		Refried Beans			
Whole Grain (WG) Bread	Cornbread or Bread Choice Brown Rice	Tortilla or Corn Shell Flatbread, or Cinn Roll or Stick	Bread Option	Roll Macaroni and Cheese	Hamburger Bun or Slider Bun
Extras			Jello		

206

	Monday	Tuesday	Wednesday	Thursday	Friday
Week 2					
Meat	Chicken Poppers—Sweet and Sour or Plain	Pigs in a Blanket or Hot Dog or Corn Dog (Turkey Frank)	Chicken Wrap, Cheese Chicken Quesadilla, Cheese	Meat Sauce or Breezy Beefy Mac or Lasagna	Grilled Cheese
Fruit	Fresh Fruit Choice	Fresh Fruit Choice or Fruit Crisp	Fresh or Canned Fruit	Canned Fruit Choice	Fresh or Canned Fruit Choice
Vegetables	Carrot Sticks or Rounds Celery Sticks, Cauliflower or Fresh Squash	Raw Broccoli	Salsa Corn	Salad Green Beans	Potato Rounds, Wedges or Fries
Legumes		Baked Beans			
Whole Grain (WG) Bread	Bread Fried Rice or Rice w/ Gravy	School-made Wrap or Bun or Corn Dog Wrap	Tortilla	Bread Option, Dough for Meat Pocket, or Spaghetti or Elbow	Sliced Bread
Extras			Jello	WG Brownie	

continues

Table 7–1. *continued*

	Monday	Tuesday	Wednesday	Thursday	Friday
Week 3					
Meat	Meat Loaf, Salisbury Steak, Shepherds Pie, Steak Fingers, or Sloppy Joe or Chicken	Chicken Tender	Tacos or Taco Salad (Beef or Chicken) with Cheese	Chicken Sauce Picante, or Fettuccini, or Turkey, Roast Pork or Hot Roast Beef Po Boy	Hamburger or Sliders or Chicken Pattie or Sliders Ham/Cheese (choice of 2 sand)
Fruit	Fresh Fruit Choice	Fresh Fruit Choice	Fresh Fruit Choice	Canned Fruit Choice	Fresh or Canned Fruit Choice
Vegetables	Raw Broccoli or Potatoes, Mashed w/ or w/o Gravy or Corn	Salad	Green Leaf Lettuce Salsa	Carrot Sticks or Rounds Celery Sticks, Cauliflower or Fresh Squash	Potato Rounds, Wedges or Fries, Green Leaf Lettuce
Legumes		Baked Beans	Pinto Beans or Black Beans		
Whole Grain (WG) Bread	Roll or Bun or Bread Option and Corn Chips	Bread Option Macaroni and Cheese	Tortilla or Corn Shell Tacos Cinn. Stick and Corn Chips Taco Salad	Bread Option or Po Boy Brown Rice or WG Pasta	Hamburger Bun
Extras	Oatmeal Cookie			Jello	

208

	Monday	Tuesday	Wednesday	Thursday	Friday
Week 4					
Meat	Meat Sauce or Hot Meat Pocket or Breezy Beefy Mac	Chicken Nugget or Tenders	Pig in a Blanket/ Hot Dog or Ham/ Cheese or Salad Supreme	Chicken-Oven Fried, Baked or BBQ or Pork Roast or Turkey Roast	Pizza or Mozzarella Stick or Chicken Quesadilla
Fruit	Fresh Fruit Choice	Fresh or Canned Fruit Choice	Fresh Fruit Choice	Canned Fruit Choice	Fresh or Canned Fruit Choice
Vegetables	Salad Green Beans	Raw Broccoli Potatoes w/ or w/o gravy	Salad Baked Potato or Sweet Potato Corn/Bean Salsa	Carrot Sticks or Rounds	Marinara or Salsa Corn
Legumes			Baked Beans	Black Eyed Peas or Red Beans	
Whole Grain (WG) Bread	Dough for Meat Pocket, Bread Options, or Pasta/ Spaghetti or Elbow	Bread Option	Sliced Bread Option or School-made Wrap or Bun Bread Option	Biscuit Brown Rice	Tortilla Pizza Crust or Mozzarella Stick Bread
Extras	Oatmeal Cookie			Jello	Breadstick with Mozzarella only

209

The swallowing and feeding team case manager is responsible for the following:

- Meeting with the cafeteria manager to design the student's monthly meal calendars that are in compliance with the student's individual swallowing and feeding plan and the regulations by the Federal Register for school lunch programs
- Working with the cafeteria staff to set up a food alteration station in the cafeteria, which includes a blender or processor for pureeing food
- Training classroom staff to prepare the food according to the recommendations on the student's swallowing and feeding plan
- Monitoring texture modifications and cafeteria meal trays periodically to ensure that the student's food is being prepared correctly

The school cafeteria manager will be responsible for the following:

- Ensuring that the food presented on the student's meal tray follows the individual monthly meal calendar, which was determined in collaboration with the swallowing and feeding case manager and that the food offered can be modified according to the student's swallowing and feeding plan
- Setting up a blending station when needed for the alteration of foods according to the child's swallowing and feeding plan
- Providing for the sterilization of the materials used in the blending station

The school cafeteria worker is responsible for the following:

- Following the student's individualized menu, substituting meal items when indicated to ensure that the student's tray matches the monthly meal menu changes
- Maintaining the blending station in the cafeteria, including the cleaning of the blender and its parts

The classroom personnel will be responsible for the following:

- Modifying the food textures according to the provisions in the child's swallowing and feeding plan

- Modifying liquids according to the provisions in the child's swallowing and feeding plan
- Feeding children with swallowing and feeding plans who are unable to self-feed
- Overseeing and monitoring children who self-feed according to the directives in their swallowing and feeding plan

Often the classroom assistant or paraprofessional will be responsible for preparing the student's tray for breakfast and lunch; however, it is ultimately the responsibility of the classroom teacher to ensure that the student's meal is prepared correctly.

Providing a nutritious meal at school that meets the requirements of the student's swallowing and feeding plan is a team effort. It is essential that team members understand their role in ensuring that the child's diet is appropriate. It is the responsibility of the swallowing and feeding team case manager to oversee this process, including ongoing monitoring of all personnel involved.

Designing a Special Diet in a School Cafeteria

The first step in meeting the mealtime needs of a student who is being followed by the swallowing and feeding team is for the team to write a plan for the student that addresses each of his or her individual needs. This plan then must be implemented during the student's school day. The first step in modifying the student's cafeteria meal is to meet with the school cafeteria manager and review the monthly meal calendar replacing foods that cannot be altered with foods that will meet the student's plan. For example, the lunch program is having pizza on Tuesday and the student needs his food pureed; the cafeteria manager substitutes chicken on the days that pizza is on the menu. The cafeteria staff saves and freezes foods that can be pureed for students allowing them to substitute these foods for others that the student cannot have (Box 7–1 and Box 7–2).

Setting Up a Food Alteration Station in the Cafeteria

In order for the classroom staff to blend and puree foods or to mechanically alter it, the cafeteria will need a blending station that is assessable to the classroom staff preparing the student's meals. This station usually has a bullet type blender with various

Box 7–1. Swallowing and Feeding Team Diet Preparation Procedure

1. It is determined that the student needs to have a diet modification. The 6-dysphagia diets are puree, mechanically chopped, minced, ground, chopped, and modified regular foods.
2. If the child's swallowing and feeding plan indicates a diet that requires that the food be altered prior to putting it on the tray (e.g., puree, mechanically chopped, minced, or ground) then a diet order should be obtained from the student's physician stating the required food consistency. Have the physician fill out the *Prescription of School Meal Modification Form* found in Appendix G. A copy should be given to the cafeteria manager and swallowing and feeding team case manager.
3. Swallowing and feeding case manager should talk to the cafeteria manager about the needs of the student.
4. Cafeteria manager will contact the food service director to determine on a case-by-case basis if a meeting is necessary to adapt the school menu.
5. If the student needs a puree diet and the school does not have a food processor, contact the swallowing and feeding team administrator to get a food processor for the school.
6. Once a meeting occurs (with the cafeteria manager and/ or the food service director) then a station should be set up in the cafeteria with the food processor.
7. The classroom staff will be responsible for:
   a. Preparing the food presented on the student's tray according to the swallowing and feeding plan.
   b. Rinsing the food processor (bullet) after use
8. The cafeteria staff will be responsible for:
   a. Sanitizing the food processor on a daily basis
   b. Adjusting portion sizes of food as necessary
   c. Changing food items as necessary
   d. Providing additional liquid as needed (milk, broth, juice)
9. A new diet order should be obtained each year and a copy given to the cafeteria manager at the school and the swallowing and feeding team administrator.

Box 7–2. Menu Guidelines/Suggestions

Cafeteria Manager will work with classroom staff to determine what foods the student tolerates. Use the following guidelines until the swallowing and feeding case manager suggests otherwise:

1. Omit breads (rolls, taco shells, corn chips). Substitute rice, cornbread, macaroni, spaghetti
2. Use chocolate milk to puree brownies, cookies
3. Use juice to puree fruits
4. Use broth to puree meat
5. Remove skin from meats
6. Omit most raw vegetables (lettuce, carrots, broccoli, cauliflower, squash, celery, etc.)
7. Omit cooked vegetables that do not puree well, such as corn
8. Cook and freeze individual portions of chicken, beef, meat sauce, red beans, and so forth to substitute for pizza or other items not tolerated

Food service will not purchase items not normally on bid. Any foods sent from home must be kept in an area other than the school kitchen and prepared by classroom staff.

---

size containers so that the staff members can modify the foods presented on the student's tray within the cafeteria kitchen. In order to comply with sanitary guidelines, food alteration should always occur in the cafeteria kitchen and not in a student's classroom.

The tray is brought to the blending station with the student's individualized meal and the classroom staff adapts each food item for the child and places it back on the cafeteria tray. Once all of the foods are ready, the classroom staff member brings the tray out to the student in the cafeteria where the child is able to eat with all of the other students. Following this preparation, the school staff rinses out the containers used and the cafeteria staff members wash the blender and its parts and leave it set up for the next meal. This process ensures that the student's meal is prepared under sanitary conditions, that the processor is sterilized, and that, when possible, the student is able to eat with his or her peers.

Parent/Guardian Provided Meals

In many cases the parents/guardians of students with swallowing and feeding concerns will prefer to provide their child's meals from home. When the parents/guardians decide to provide the meal from home, it must meet the requirements of the student's swallowing and feeding plan at school. While parents/guardians are free to make decisions on how they feed their children at home, the school district is required to follow the district swallowing and feeding team's recommendations for safe eating at school that is spelled out in the Swallowing and Feeding Plan (see Appendix B).

Information Sharing With Parents/Guardians

When a child has a swallowing and feeding plan at school, the school team should meet with the parents to inform them of the findings of their swallowing and feeding evaluation and their recommendations. As stated previously, the parents/guardians are part of the problem-solving team responsible for determining how the student is fed. Once the plan is written, the parents/guardians should be trained on how their child will be fed at school and informed of the types of foods and textures that the child may eat at school. Parents/guardians may have questions about the types of foods that can be pureed or mechanically chopped. They may want to know if they are responsible for altering the food or if the school team can adapt the food sent. In many cases, the parents are already providing the student with foods that meet the plan. The school team may be able to offer them some other options or different foods that could be given to their child. Consulting with parents on their child's special feeding needs will help them to provide more nutritious meals at home and to pack a lunch for their child that has appropriate foods for school. They also need to be informed of the district's responsibility to ensure their child's safety at school; therefore, some foods sent from home may need to be altered to meet the recommendations of the swallowing and feeding team and the student's plan. In most cases, parents/guardians agree with the plan and adhere to the diet prescribed; however, in some cases, parents/guardians insist on sending foods that, in the district team's professional opinion, the student cannot safely tolerate. In those cases, the district must follow the district's swallowing and feeding plan. Legally, the district must ensure that the student is safe at school. This highlights the importance of having a strong, positive working relationship with the student's parents/guardians.

Training School Staff to Prepare Special Diets

In many cases, students will need to have their meals altered either in food or liquid consistency, amount of food per bite, positioning, and food-to-drink presented ratio. This requires that the swallowing and feeding team case manager train all of the classroom staff, including alternates in the event the main feeder is absent, on how to safely prepare a student's meal and feed the student. Regardless of whether the student's meal is from the cafeteria or parent/guardian prepared, the classroom staff must ensure that the food is prepared according to the student's plan.

The case manager demonstrates for the classroom staff the recommended consistency of the food being prepared and the viscosity of the liquids. Each staff member needs to practice and demonstrate competency in preparing the student's meal. According to ASHA (2015), diet modifications consist of altering the viscosity, texture, temperature, or taste of a food or liquid to facilitate safety and ease of swallowing. Typical modifications include thickening thin liquids or softening, chopping, or pureeing solid foods. Taste or temperature of a food may be altered to provide additional sensory input for swallowing. Thickening agents, which may be used to prepare nectar, honey, or pudding thickness for liquid, are usually provided by the parents but may also be provided by the school system. Altering the viscosity of a liquid presents challenges with all populations with dysphagia. SLPs working in school systems have the responsibility to keep up with the latest research and information on the best protocols for thickening liquids for children with pharyngeal phase dysphagia. The goal is for the student to eat as normal a diet as is considered safe by the school swallowing and feeding team based on their evaluation of the student's swallowing and feeding skills as well as the student's medical history and condition.

Once the classroom staff has demonstrated that they can consistently prepare the student's meals according to the recommendations on the swallowing and feeding plan, they verify their training and agree to follow the plan by signing their name, position, and date of training on the plan. This is essential because a swallowing and feeding plan is only effective if it is followed with fidelity. Ultimately, it is the responsibility of the classroom teacher that the plan is implemented correctly.

The School District's Swallowing and Feeding Team's Role With Nutrition

The primary responsibility for a child's overall nutrition lies with his or her parents/guardians. Children must be adequately nourished and hydrated in order to actively participate in school and in their curriculum. The district swallowing and feeding team works with children who have been identified with dysphagia or significant behavioral/sensory feeding disorders to ensure that they receive adequate nutrition and hydration at school by monitoring their status and ensuring that they are fed safely and efficiently. Children with dysphagia as the result of a developmental disability, neurological disorder (e.g., cerebral palsy, traumatic brain injury), genetic syndromes, behavioral factors (e.g., food refusal or selectivity), and complex medical conditions (e.g., gastroesophageal reflux disorder or pulmonary disease) are at high risk for developing undernutrition and/or dehydration. Children who are on restrictive diets as a result of severe or multiple food allergies, autism, or food intolerance should be observed and monitored for nutritional deficiencies (Arvedson, Delanedy, Fischer, & Kirby, 2008). The district team designs a swallowing and feeding plan that ensures that the student is fed properly at school and is participating in his or her meals at school.

When there is a concern that the student is not receiving adequate nutrition and hydration, the school team should work with parents and physicians to determine the causes and solutions to the undernourishment and dehydration. In some cases, a student may appear to be severely undernourished or dehydrated and the parents/guardians do not respond to the concerns reported by the school staff. It is the obligation of the school personnel, as mandatory reporters, to report the student's condition to the Office of Protective Services when parents are unresponsive and the child is in a serious condition. School districts work closely with parents/guardians to foster trust and well-being; however, in some cases, the district will not be successful and must act in the interest of the child (National Health Service, 2013a).

Undernutrition and Dehydration in Students With Swallowing and Feeding Disorders

Malnutrition is typically described as the condition that occurs when the body does not get the right amount of vitamins, minerals, and other nutrients it needs to maintain healthy tissues and organ function. It can be in the form of undernutrition or overnutrition. In schools, undernutrition is more common; however, children with behavioral feeding disorders often consume large quantities of calories with little nutritional value. Therefore, the school team should be aware of this risk, especially with that population. In both cases, the student's diet lacks the nutrients needed for growth and health (National Health Service, 2013b).

   Any professional working in the area of swallowing and feeding should be familiar with the signs and symptoms of undernutrition and dehydration. In the school setting, most students are not sick, nor are they monitored daily by medical personnel. As a result, the responsibility for identifying when a child is suffering from a nutrition or hydration concern may lay with the student's family and the school team: primarily the SLP, OT, nurse, and classroom teacher. According to the Johns Hopkins Children's Center website, chronic undernutrition occurs in approximately 1% of children in the United States. Children who are chronically undernourished may be short for their age, thin, bloated, and/or listless and have weakened immune systems. These deficiencies can affect any system in the body. Children who are severely undernourished may have long-term effects in language, cognition, digestive problems, and other serious medical complications including death.

Signs and Symptoms of Undernutrition

The school swallowing and feeding team members should have the training necessary to recognize the signs and symptoms of children with nutritional and/or hydration concerns. A symptom is something that a child might feel or report or may even be observable. A child may complain of a pain in their stomach or that they feel tired. A sign, on the other hand, is something that others will detect, often a physician, such as a rash or body-fat distribution. Both are important to consider when undernutrition or dehydration is suspected (National Health Service, 2013c).

Recognizing Undernutrition

The school-based staff have opportunities during the school year to notice changes in the nutritional status of the their students. Malnourished children may report that they are tired and don't feel like working. They may be irritable, anxious, and disoriented. The teacher may observe that the child bruises easily, has diarrhea, and that he or she often has rashes. The student may have achy joints and muscle twitches. If these symptoms persist, the teacher, SLP, OT, or nurse should contact the parents/guardians to discuss the student's condition. A child experiencing a thinning of their hair, loss of body composition such as body fat, hollow sunken eyes, protruding bones, and thin, dry, inelastic skin should receive medical attention immediately. These symptoms are an indication that the child may be severely undernourished.

Signs and Symptoms of Dehydration

The child with dehydration presents with a unique set of signs and symptoms. This child may have thirst, a dry, sticky mouth, decreased urine output, and few or no tears when crying. The student may be sleepy, complain of a headache, dizziness, or lightheadedness. Severe dehydration is a condition that requires immediate medical attention. The student with severe dehydration may be extremely thirsty and have a very dry mouth, skin, and mucous membranes. This child may be extremely fussy or sleepy. Their eyes may be sunken and their skin dry and inelastic. They may produce little or no urine and when they do urinate it may be very dark. The nurse may observe that the child has low blood pressure, rapid breathing, and a rapid heartbeat. If the school staff observes these signs and symptoms in a student the parents/guardians should be contacted and the child should see a physician immediately. In most cases, when the school staff is concerned about the student's nutritional status, they will work closely with the parents/guardians and the child's physician to address these concerns both at home and at school. The treatment may include altering the student's diet and food presentation. The district team is in the unique position of being able to assist parents/guardians in ensuring that their child receives adequate nutrition and hydration at school.

Training Classroom Staff to Recognize the Signs and Symptoms of Undernutrition and Dehydration

Training is an important component throughout the swallowing and feeding team procedures in the school setting. All members of the team that work with children with swallowing and feeding disorders should be trained in how to recognize the signs and symptoms of undernutrition and dehydration. The school nurse can work with the personnel in each classroom to train them to know what to look for and how to respond when they have a concern. It is important to document the training sessions, who were trained, and when they were trained. Periodic retraining is also beneficial. Table 7–2 offers a summary of the signs and symptoms of undernutrition and dehydration, which can be given to teachers and classroom assistants to refer when they have a concern.

Treatment for Undernutrition

In many cases, the school team is able to assess the student's swallowing and feeding skills and establish a swallowing and feeding plan that not only provides a way for the child to eat safely and efficiently at school but also to address nutritional issues.

Table 7–2. Signs and Symptoms of Undernutrition and Dehydration in School-Aged Children

Undernutrition	Dehydration
Mild Moderate Undernutrition	*Mild Moderate Dehydration*
• Bruises easily	• Dry sticky mouth
• Rashes, change in pigmentation	• Sleepiness/tiredness
• Achy joints	• Thirst
• Soft, tender bones	• Decreased urine output
• Gums bleed easily	• Few or no tears when crying
• Tongue swollen or shriveled and cracked	• Dry skin
• Increased sensitivity to light, night blindness	• Headache
	• Constipation
• Diarrhea	• Dizziness or lightheadedness
• Disorientation	• Reduced sweating
• Irritability, anxiety, and attention deficits	• Reduced skin elasticity
• Loss of reflexes/lack of muscular coordination	
• Muscle twitches	
• Fatigue	
• Delays in language and cognitive skills	
• Longer healing time for wounds	
• Longer recovery time from infections and illness	
Severe Undernutrition: A medical emergency	*Severe Dehydration: A medical emergency*
• Thin hair, tightly curled, and pulls out easily	• Extreme thirst
• Loss of body composition including body fat, hollow sunken eyes, protruding bones.	• Extreme fussiness or sleepiness
	• Very dry mouth, skin and mucous membranes
• Apathy or unresponsiveness	• Little or no urination—urine that is produced is dark
• Skin thin, dry, inelastic, pale, and cold.	• Sunken eyes
• If prolonged: heart, liver or respiratory failure	• Shriveled/dry skin, inelastic
	• Rapid breathing
• Slow development in children	• Rapid heartbeat
• Impaired mental function	• No tears when crying
	• Low blood pressure
	• Fever

Physicians may recommend that some children with serious undernutrition be fed using alternative methods of nutrition and hydration. A percutaneous endoscopic gastrostomy (PEG) tube may be inserted directly into the gastrointestinal track to ensure that the student receives adequate nutrition. If the child is tube fed because of undernutrition, oral feeding may continue and is recommended. Once the child's nutritional status is upgraded, the physician may decide to remove the tube and the student can continue with oral feeding. This decision is based on the medical doctor's recommendations with consultation by the registered dietician and medical SLP. Another alternative method is the nasogastric tube (NG), which may be inserted temporarily to improve the student's nutritional status. The NG tube may be used when a child is too fragile or sick to have a PEG tube inserted or when the condition is thought to be short term and a temporary solution is recommended. The child's physician is responsible for these decisions but the school nurse and school team will work closely with the medical team to ensure that the student's needs at school are being met. This may require the school nurse to be trained in NG and/or PEG tube feeding. PEG tube feeding is a trainable skill and the school nurse may train classroom staff to tube feed the students. The NG tube requires skillful insertion, typically with an X-ray to verify placement. Daily activities at school can compromise the placement of the NG tube; therefore, it is recommended that NG tube feeding only be done at school by a registered nurse, in close conjunction with the physician and parents. This may require training specific to the child and NG tube feeding.

How a School District Addresses Nutritional Concerns

When the school swallowing and feeding team is concerned that a disabled student is undernourished and/or dehydrated the Swallowing and Feeding Team Procedure described in Chapter 3 allows the team to determine if the undernutrition is the result of a swallowing and feeding disorder, medical condition, or neglect. The team works closely with the parents/guardians using the Parent/Guardian Interview Form (see Appendix D) to discuss the student's medical issues and feeding practices at home. The student is evaluated for swallowing and feeding disorders including behavioral and sensorimotor concerns. If it is determined that the child has dysphagia or a behavioral sensorimotor feeding disorder that prevents them from receiving adequate nutrition, the team writes a Swallowing and Feeding Plan (see Appendix B) ensuring that the child receives adequate nutrition and hydration at school. Classroom personnel are trained on the preparation of the student's meals and the implementation of the plan. At the same time, the team works closely with the parents-guardians and physicians to make sure that medical conditions that affect the child's ability to consume adequate calories are addressed.

When a child's health is already compromised because of inadequate nutrition and/or hydration, it is recommended that the school team work with the parents and assist them on how to safely feed their child at home. When a student continues to come to school hungry, in spite of documented attempts to provide training, or if the student does not have a feeding disorder, which is responsible for the lack of nutrition, then the district may suspect neglect and therefore has a responsibility to report the concern to the Office of Child Protective Services. Each state has an agency that is responsible for taking calls from concerned individuals regarding child abuse and neglect. The name of this agency varies from state to state; however, their function and purpose is the same. Educators, by law, are required to report any suspected cases of child abuse or neglect. Follow your district's guidelines for reporting to protective services; however, ultimately the responsibility lies with the person observing the concern.

Student Profile: Undernutrition

John was a severely impaired cerebral palsy, high school student in a severe profound class placement. The swallowing and feeding team in junior high school did not follow him. John, for the first time, did not attend the extended school year program during the summer, and when he started at the new high school he was extremely thin. When the school nurse weighed him, he was 65 pounds. He was immediately referred to the swallowing and feeding team and the procedure was followed. John's mother participated minimally in the process. A swallowing and feeding plan was established based on the information that the team had at that time. John had the signs and symptoms of undernourishment: lethargy, dry skin, minimal urination, and thin hair. The school team was not sure of the cause of his nutrition deficits and wanted to ensure that pharyngeal dysphagia was not responsible for his limited food intake. In addition, the fact that he only attended school two to three days a week complicated the process. The teacher had a journal that went back and forth from home, which seemed to be the most effective way of communicating with the mother. John's mother was not interested in taking him for an MBSS and did not respond to requests for a physician referral.

A pattern emerged where, when John was at school, he consumed many calories in the form of puree foods and enriched milkshakes. He responded positively to the meals and, although he was nonverbal, he often signaled at school that he wanted to eat by pointing to his watch. He ate throughout the day when at school. However, then he would miss a few days at school and come back lethargic. The mother eventually agreed to a swallow study and the swallowing and feeding case manager and administrator accompanied the mother and John to the study. The outcome from the study indicated that John had a functioning pharyngeal swallow, weak oral mechanism and functioning, and a puree diet with thin liquids was recommended. The results of this study supported the suspicions of the school team that there was neglect going on at home. A referral to protective services was made. John continued at school on the enriched puree diet and was eventually placed in a home for severely involved adolescents. The school team was pleased with his change in living conditions as his new home provided him with consistent meals as well as proper hygiene care and other needs.

Monitoring a Student's Nutrition Status

Once it has been determined that a child has undernutrition or dehydration and the presenting problems have been addressed, the swallowing and feeding team should monitor the student's nutritional status. Keeping a daily food log on the foods and liquids that a child consumes can be helpful. This log should include the types of foods, amount offered and amount consumed, as well as liquids offered and consumed. The classroom teacher should be responsible for maintaining the log and the log should be reviewed by the swallowing and feeding case manager and the school nurse (School-Based Swallowing and Feeding Team Daily Feeding Log, see Appendix K). Once the student's weight is stabilized and he or she is getting adequate nutrition, the logs no longer need to be kept. In addition, the school nurse can weigh students with nutritional concerns on a regular schedule to monitor their weight. This can be a challenge for children who are in wheelchairs or who are unable to support their own weight. It may require a school staff member weighing himself or herself first without holding the student and then while holding the student. In some cases, because of the size of the student and the student's condition, weighing him or her at school may not be possible. The school swallowing and feeding team may be able to work with parents for the student to be periodically weighed at the doctor's office.

Cultural Considerations

The United States is becoming increasingly more diverse. There is an increase in citizens who are non-European and who come with different cultures, languages, and customs. According to Davis-McFarland (2008), culture is the filter through which people view the world and evaluate all aspects of their existence. It is extremely important in the public school system, when working with parents/guardians on food and feeding, that the district team is knowledgeable and respectful of the family's beliefs and customs. Davis-McFarland recommends that the school team take the time to work with families to determine appropriate diet recommendations at school. The Parental/Guardian Interview Form (see Appendix D) provides an avenue for the swallowing and feeding case manager to review with the parents/guardians preferred foods and dietary practices in the home. This allows for the team to be sensitive to food beliefs within the culture of the family and to make recommendations that respect those beliefs while at the same time providing a plan that ensures the child is fed safely at school and receives adequate nutrition and hydration. Working closely with the parents/guardians when evaluating a student's swallowing and feeding and then writing a plan facilitates a better and more workable plan that has the support of the family and therefore a better chance to be successful.

Summary of Addressing Nutrition in the School Setting

Nutrition and hydration are at the basis of swallowing and feeding. In order for students to access their curriculum, participate socially, and attend school they must have adequate nutrition and hydration. Swallowing and feeding team members should be familiar with the School Lunch Program and how it provides free and low cost meals to students. They can work with cafeteria staff members to provide a diet at school that will meet the recommendations of the student's swallowing and feeding plan. Getting students with swallowing and feeding concerns to be adequately nourished at school will require a team effort to modify monthly meal menus, set up a blending station in the cafeteria, alter foods, and safely feed students. In cases where students bring a lunch from home, the team will need to work closely with parents to ensure that the meal meets the recommendations of the student's swallowing and feeding plan.

It is essential that the team members be able to recognize the signs and symptoms of undernutrition and dehydration and to identify a student who is at risk. School team members need to work closely with families and physicians to meet the specific nutritional needs of the students. Classroom personnel and swallowing and feeding team members should be trained to identify when a student's nutritional status is compromised. With all students, it is important to take into consideration a family's cultural customs and beliefs in regard to food and mealtimes. This helps the parents/guardians to accept the recommendations and to work with the school team.

References

American Speech-Language-Hearing Association. (2015). *Clinical topics: Pediatric dysphagia.* Retrieved from http://www.asha.com

Arvedson, J., Delaney, A., Fischer, E., & Kirby, M., (2008). *Let's eat: Pediatric nutrition, behavioral, and oral sensorimotor issues.* 2008 ASHA Convention Handouts, Chicago, IL.

Davis-McFarland, E. (2008). Family and cultural issues in a school swallowing and feeding program. *Language, Speech, and Hearing Services in Schools, 39,* 199–213.

Department of Agriculture Food and Nutrition Service; Nutrition Standards in the National School Lunch and School Breakfast Programs, 77 Fed. Reg. (January 26, 2012) (to be codified at 7, C.F.R. pts. 210 & 220).

Gunderson, G. (2014). *National school lunch program early programs by states.* Retrieved from http://www.fns.usda.gov/nslp/history

National Health Service. (2013a). *Causes of malnutrition.* Retrieved from http://www.nhs.uk/Conditions/Malnutrition/Pages/Causes.aspx

National Health Service. (2013b). *Malnutrition.* Retrieved from http://www.nhs.uk/conditions/Malnutrition/Pages/Introduction.aspx

National Health Service. (2013c). *Symptoms of malnutrition.* Retrieved from http://www.nhs.uk/Conditions/Malnutrition/Pages/Symptoms.aspx

United States Department of Agriculture. (2014). *National school lunch program.* Retrieved from http://www.fns.usda.gov/nslp/history_2

8

Working With Parents/Guardians of Students With Swallowing and Feeding Disorders in the School Setting

Emily M. Homer

Introduction: A Personal Perspective

October 24, 1963, President John F. Kennedy signed the Maternal and Child Health and Mental Retardation Planning Amendment to the Social Security Act, which was the first major legislation to combat mental illness and retardation. With the passage of this legislation, life for children with disabilities was about to improve and with it the life of their parents and family. Another legislation was approved on October 31, 1963 that provided funding for the construction of facilities related to the prevention, care, and treatment of people with intellectual disabilities. Joseph was 7 years old at the time. Up to the point when he was born in 1956, my sister and I had a typical family experience for that time. I am not sure of my first memory or knowledge that he was different because, to me, he was my brother and I loved him completely. His birth into my family changed the life of my parents and my entire family. My parents had their own business, which required both of them to work. Prior to the 1963 legislation, he was home all day with a sitter. He could not talk, was not toilet trained, and was frequently ill. There was nowhere for him to go to school to learn and you rarely saw children like my brother in the stores or out in public. After the 1963 legislation, my parents were contacted regarding the opening of a new school for children like Joseph and they wanted him to attend the first class of its kind. This significantly enriched his life and provided some help for my parents.

My family adjusted as best as they could to life with a disabled child, but to an outsider, some of the decisions my parents made may have been difficult to understand. Many times our household was in a panic because of a sudden high fever, with my parents having to rely on extended family to help them. I recall my mother being so exhausted, at times, that she came home and collapsed in her bed after work. She would be up during the night with my brother who didn't always sleep at night. As I got older, I was my brother's sitter and, eventually, so were my friends. The teacher's and paraprofessionals who worked with Joseph also became sitters. They were lifesavers, allowing my parents to go on vacations. We were fortunate because my parents could afford childcare, high medical bills, and lived near extended family. Many families are not in that position.

In most cases, parents and families do the best they can to meet the needs of their disabled child while at the same time raising their other children, supporting the family, and achieving a quality of life. As a school team working with families, we have the information that is presented to us. We will not always know all of the details and we may have more questions than answers. In many cases, the information that we do not have may be very important in understanding how the family is functioning. By working closely with families and gaining their trust, we have a better chance of achieving our goal of helping our students be healthy and safe at school and able to learn and participate in their curriculum.

Raising a Child With a Swallowing and Feeding Disorder

The goal of this chapter is to provide some thoughts and insights into some of the issues families go through when there is a child in the family with disabilities, including swallowing and feeding disorders. Suggestions of what school district teams can do to help parents/guardians are also addressed. While this chapter offers considerations when trying to understand the perspective of parents/guardians, it is not possible for anyone to completely understand what families go through or how they react to their situation. Each family deals with the challenges and rewards of living with a child with a disability in their own way and no one can presume to know how they feel or how they should feel or act.

Educators try hard to do what is best for children and their families within the context of the school setting. "Working with students who have dysphagia can certainly be difficult, but understanding families' perspectives can prove not only helpful, but, in many instances, crucial to developing and implementing effective programming" (Angell, Bailey, Nicholson, & Stoner, 2009, p. 10).

Family Issues and Concerns Related to Raising a Child With a Swallowing and Feeding Disorder

Typically, parents/guardians have hopes and dreams for their children both before and after their birth. When a child is born with or develops a disability, the future is frequently an unknown, as are expectations for that child. Stages and developmental milestones that are considered a normal part of having a child are different for a child with a disability. These differences affect all aspects of family life. School-based professionals should work toward developing an appreciation of the impact that having a child with a developmental disability can have on the family and develop sensitivity for the complexities that families with disabled children face (Handleman, 1995).

Many studies have looked at stress factors in families of children with multiple disabilities. According to Brown & Bhavnagri (1996), many of these studies state that parents of disabled children report higher levels of stress than parents without disabled children. Lopez, Clifford, Minnes, and Ouellette-Kuntz, (2008) compared the stress levels of parents of preschool developmentally delayed children with parents of preschoolers without disabilities. They found that parents of children with developmental delays experienced higher levels of stress. This stress was increased when the issues were related to their child's delayed development and/or specific diagnosis. It may be helpful to go through some of the issues and concerns that families of children with disabilities in general and swallowing and feeding disorders specifically may experience.

Medical Concerns

Many children with swallowing and feeding disorders in the school setting have multiple disabilities and may be classified as moderate or severely disabled. These children may have cerebral palsy, Down syndrome, genetic disorders, or other neurological disorders. In addition to concerns about the child's ability to get nutrition, the parents are faced with serious medical conditions that are unique for each child. For example, children with cerebral palsy have other complications such as motor control, balance, seizure disorders, hearing and vision impairments, and digestive issues. Children with Down syndrome are more likely to have heart defects and be prone more to infections than their typical peers. They may have epilepsy, digestive issues, and spinal defects. These multiple health concerns are not limited to children with cerebral palsy or Down syndrome, but they offer an example of the many medical issues that parents may be facing while at the same time trying to manage school placement as well as their child's swallowing and feeding disorders.

Children with significant disabilities frequently spend their early years in and out of hospitals and clinics. The family adapts itself to these episodes and they become part of the family's normal lifestyle. While it may become normal, it is never routine. There is no predicting when a child will start experiencing difficulty, when a child will need emergency care or when a family faces the fear of a serious illness and hospitalization. These frequent interactions, with what for other families are rare occasions, can place additional stress on all members of the family and the extended family. Grandparents, aunts, and uncles may be called on to stay with siblings while the parents/guardians are at the hospital with the sick child. Siblings may miss important school and social activities such as parties, because their brother or sister is in the hospital. They may worry that their sibling will not get better and may see their parents upset. Parents want all of their children to be happy and healthy, and they stress over not being available for the other children. These episodes, while extremely difficult, often strengthen and pull a family together. It can, however, also have an opposite effect.

For example, the school team will need to be sensitive to a parent/guardian's hesitation to go to the hospital for a swallow study, which may not seem medically necessary to them. It is sometimes helpful for the school team to describe how the MBSS/VFSS is conducted and let the parents/guardians know what to expect. Informing the parents/guardians of the possible outcomes of the evaluation helps them to understand and to be more receptive to the test. For example, informing the parents that if there is a delay in the child's swallowing, we can alter how we give the child liquids by thickening them. Parents/guardians may worry that the child will need to be sedated, or that the evaluation will be invasive. Clearing up some of these fears and concerns may help them to agree to the test. There is often the fear that the school district team is trying to take away their ability to feed their child and that tube feeding will be recommended. The school team should let parents/guardians know the reasons for the referral and what the possible outcomes may be.

It is always important for the school team to work closely with the medical team and the parents. In order for the school team to communicate with the medical team, the parents need to sign a Release of Information form. Once this form is signed by the parents/guardians the school team can inform the child's physician of their concerns and the physician can share medical conditions that could affect school performance. This communication with the medical team and the parents helps with the management of the child's swallowing and feeding disorder in school and keeps the school team, medical team, and parents all on the same page.

Student Profile: Working with Parents

Kyle is a profoundly mentally disabled, elementary school student with cerebral palsy and a seizure disorder. A modified barium swallow study indicated that Kyle was safe to eat orally; however, the physician chose to insert a PEG tube because of "failure to thrive." Kyle was placed on continuous feed for two years but continued to be fed by his mother and was not fed at school. The mom was ready for the tube to be removed and for the school to increase oral feedings. A follow-up MBSS indicated that Kyle was safe for oral feeding and his weight had improved; however, the physician called in during his IEP and delayed the removal by 1 year. He wanted the student to gain additional weight before relying entirely on oral feeding. A year later the MBSS was repeated with the same results. The school team, consisting of the SLP, OT, nurse, teacher, and paraprofessional conducted an interdisciplinary observation. The student immediately began coughing, eyes watered, and he showed several signs of aspiration. The school team was not comfortable proceeding with the feeding and it was stopped. The parent was very upset and indicated that during the MBSS the student was fed in the "blue chair" where he was positioned in a safe way for feeding. The school team had failed to adequately involve the mother in the transition plan for oral feeding. The interdisciplinary observation was repeated in the "blue chair" (which is a tumble form chair that was used by mom at home) and mom demonstrated feeding during the observation. The student did extremely well and from that point on the school team worked closely with the mother to transition Kyle to oral feeding. Kyle has been orally fed since and the swallowing and feeding team learned an important lesson about working with parents from the beginning.

Financial Concerns

Finances are frequently a concern in households; however, for the family with a child with swallowing and feeding disorders, the increased medical bills, time parents/guardians need off of work, and the specialized sitters, equipment, and therapies add to these concerns. While school district personnel cannot assist parents with financial concerns, they should be aware of the possible strains it can put on a family. Districts may refer parents to organizations and state resources that can assist them. One way that the swallowing and feeding team can help parents/ guardians is to inform them ahead of time that referrals from the school team for instrumental testing such as the MBSS/VFSS are the responsibility of the district. This will relieve any concerns about the costs related to this test.

Concerns for the Future

The future for families with disabled children can be an area of uncertainty. Parents/guardians often have concerns about who will take care of the child when they are no longer able to care for them. Once the child is 22 and has completed school, they may worry about who will care for the adult child while they work. The child with swallowing and feeding disorders may need help at mealtimes and whenever he or she is eating, which would require a caretaker throughout the day. Parents/ guardians frequently worry about the child's health as he or she ages and/or the regression that sometimes occurs. These fears may result in the belief that their child should receive as many services as they possibly can through the school district before the child ages out. It is helpful for the school team to have an understanding of the parent/guardian's point of reference when working with their child.

School teams will need to stay focused on what is in the best interest of the child, keeping in mind that the parents may have a different opinion and perspective. There are times when more services for students are not the best or most appropriate services. School teams will need to support their recommendations with evidenced-based research and data while validating the parent/guardian's opinions.

School systems have a responsibility to help parents navigate the transition from school to home and work. When students reach a certain age level their IEP includes a transition plan. This plan is designed to help the parents and the students look at their future goals. School districts frequently have booklets, information fairs, and community outreach to assist parents/

guardians in planning for the time when their child no longer is able to attend school.

As children get older, they typically move on and become independent. Many parents/guardians look forward to the day when they have some time to themselves. Raising a child with a significant disability often means that these parents/guardians will never have their own independence from children. They may worry that, as they get older, it will be more difficult for them to care for their special needs child. These concerns for the future add stress to a family and can result in depression and anxiety. Gallagher, Phillips, Oliver, and Carroll (2008) investigated symptoms of depression and anxiety and their origins in parents caring for intellectually disabled children relative to parents of typically developing children. They found that parents of children with intellectual disabilities were more prone to depression and anxiety because of poorer sleep quality and a significantly higher caregiver burden score. The burden scale used included feeling of embarrassment and guilt, a sense of entrapment, resentment, and the experience of loss and isolation from society.

Toll on Family Structure

Mealtimes are often the times that families spend together to catch up on the day and to interact with each other. A child with a swallowing and feeding disorder can upset the family mealtime routine. There is often stress related to feeding a child with dysphagia or with behavioral feeding disorders, and this stress can carryover to the entire family. Frequently, children with feeding disorders are fed separately from the family so the parents/guardians are preparing two meals. One parent may be with the child with the feeding disorder and the other is with the rest of the family.

Eating out as a family is often a reward for school performance, a celebration, or a time for family fun. The child with a swallowing and/or feeding disorder often has difficulty eating in restaurants and may need to pack a special diet. The family may not be able to go or may be hesitant to participate in school picnics, soccer game pizza nights, or other activities in which their other children are involved. Families often adjust to these differences and end up successfully juggling both; however, it is beneficial for school personnel to be aware of the complicated lives that the families of their students live.

Student Profile: Helping a Family

Lesley was a 4-year-old student in our preschool program that was diagnosed as "failure to thrive." When she started in the school district she was on an overnight continuous tube feeding. She had a functional swallow and she needed to be weaned from the tube and return to oral feedings. The SLP, who served as the swallowing and feeding case manager, worked closely with the parents to accomplish this goal. The SLP collaborated with the student's physician to establish a plan for weaning from the tube. At Lesley's IEP meeting, the SLP discussed with the parents the importance of changing the tube feeding schedule to occur after the oral feeds, instead of the continuous feeding to which they were accustomed. She discussed with the parents how to get Lesley on the family's mealtime schedule as well as on the school mealtime schedule. The SLP recommended that Lesley sit at the table (something she had never done) both at school and at home. She enjoyed the social setting and parents were grateful for the guidance of the school team with the transition. Lesley now sits across from other students and is eating orally both at home and school.

Siblings

Typical children who grow up in homes with disabled siblings may react in completely different ways within the same family. Some siblings assume a caretaker role, taking the disabled child everywhere and playing with them constantly. Others may feel embarrassment or be unsure how to let their friends know about their sibling. Each child will react in their own way and will have their own unique relationship with the disabled sibling. Some siblings may resent the added stress on their parents and may feel that they are missing out on attention. Managing the family dynamics is another added dimension that parents/guardians of disabled children experience, and that may add stress to their situation.

Emotional Issues Related to Raising a Child With a Disability

Gallagher, Phillips, Oliver, and Carroll (2008) found that the symptoms of depression and anxiety in parents caring for intellectually disabled children were highly prevalent and that the negative psychosocial consequences of caregiving were predictive of depression, but guilt was the main emotion associated with parent's anxiety. Caring for a special needs child is complex and may result in parents, particularly mothers, having a limited social life, and it may affect their ability to work outside the home. These restrictions can result in depression and in some cases anxiety. Studies also indicated that parents of children with intellectual disabilities who report feelings of guilt also indicated a lack in confidence in their ability to parent their special needs children.

Parents/guardians typically accept the responsibility of feeding their children with joy and pride. One of the primary responsibilities of parenting is to nourish your child so that they grow into healthy adults. When a child is unable to accept the food offered by his or her parents/guardians or refuses to accept the food, it can be a very stressful thing for both the parents and the child. Parents/guardians may feel responsible for their child's undernutrition or food refusal. This associative guilt may result in an increase in parental anxiety. Working with the parents on solutions to the child's feeding issues may help parents/guardians to feel less anxious about mealtimes and, as a result, have a more positive experience (Garro, Thurman, Kerwin, & Ducette, 2005).

Parents/guardians may associate the school-based swallowing and feeding team with the fear that their child may not be able to continue to eat orally. In many cases, there is little or no risk that the child will need tube feeding, but the fear of this outcome may compromise the relationship the parents/guardians have with the school team. In many cases, eating is the last "normal" thing the child can do from the parent's perspective. They may not be able to walk, talk, or do the other things that their typical peers can do. The team will need to reassure the parents and to inform them of why their child is being evaluated and the purpose and plan of the program.

What a District Team Can Do to Help Parents

Helping Parents/Guardians to Understand Their Child's Swallowing and Feeding Disorder

A school-based swallowing and feeding team can work closely with parents to help them to understand and adapt to having a child with a swallowing and feeding disorder. They should prepare and share information with them that is driven by the evaluation and personal interactions, which reflects their child's individual needs. The team can provide illustrations and explanations that will give the parents/guardians an understanding of the anatomy and physiology related to their child's disorders. Research supports that parenting stress is reduced when parents/guardians learn about their child's medical problems and conditions (Garro et al., 2005; Horn, Feldman, & Ploof, 1995).

The school-based swallowing and feeding team can help to educate parents on their child's disorder by defining a swallowing and feeding disorder, it's signs and symptoms and how they relate to the child's disorder. Team members such as the SLP, OT, or nurse, can consult with the parents/guardians to educate them on ways that they can prevent additional complications of the child's swallowing and feeding disorder. This includes teaching them how to prepare the student's meal according to the recommended swallowing and feeding plan and helping them to learn the signs and symptoms of undernutrition and dehydration and how to react to them. When discussing with parents the recommendation of the school system's team on how to feed their child, the team must be sensitive to the parent's/ guardian's knowledge and expertise with their child and present it in a nonthreatening manner (Box 8–1).

In addition, team members can share with parents/guardians the therapeutic techniques they are using that are effective in treating their child's oral sensorimotor disorder. They can train parents/guardians to do oral sensorimotor exercises and techniques to improve oral motor skills such as chewing and to desensitize the student to new and different tastes and textures.

Box 8–1. Parent Perspective #1

Mother of a Preschool Student With Significant Swallowing and Feeding Issues Due to Cerebral Palsy

During an interview on her experience with the swallowing and feeding team at her child's school, the parent shared these thoughts:

Interviewer: How did the swallowing and feeding team help you with the transition from home to school for your preschool child?

Mother: The dysphagia team, they were excellent. They really helped a lot. Not only transitioning from home to school but even transitioning, I mean, in what he ate and what I fed him, or as texture-wise goes. We were really nervous about him starting school and having to be fed by somebody else. That was an issue; he was on puree foods. But once he got here, Ms. Patty (SLP) put a plan together and worked with the teachers and the paraprofessionals. They had him eating whole foods in no time. I don't think they know this, but they were giving him whole foods way before I was. I was scared to death to do that. I was thinking about this last night. If they hadn't pushed whole foods, he might still be on a puree diet.

Interviewer: What advice would you give therapists working with children with swallowing and feeding problems?

Mother: I wonder if they could almost do notes, even, jot down what the speech therapist is doing during the day. Jot down in the child's folder what they worked on that day so the parents can maybe reinforce the same things. A back and forth communication.

Ongoing, Regular Communication With Parents/Guardians

Regular communication with parents/guardians will keep them informed of their child's feeding status at school and progress in feeding or oral sensorimotor therapy. In addition, this communication will help to reduce stress and concern regarding how their child is doing at school. Family and school team interaction consisting of open communication is essential in addressing swallowing and feeding in a school setting. It is important for school-based teams to foster a sense of partnership with the parents/guardians that consists of consistent communication. Communication with parents can be in the form of notebook entries that go back and forth from school to home, e-mails, phone calls, and periodic face-to-face conferences (Angell et al., 2009; Homer, 2008).

Parents/guardians provide the school team with invaluable knowledge about their child regarding feeding at home, medical history, cultural considerations, and personality characteristics while the school team serves as a support and an information source (Homer, 2008). The swallowing and feeding team procedure includes having the parents/guardians participate from the very beginning as part of the problem-solving team. They should be involved and informed throughout the process.

Validate the Parents/Guardians Perspective

There are ways that school swallowing and feeding team members can work with parents that validates their feelings, emotions, and opinions and still provides the services the student needs to be fed safely and efficiently at school. From the beginning of the team's interaction with the family, it is important to relay the message that the parent's/guardian's experience and knowledge of their child is valued. The parents/guardians have a history with their child that provides the team with invaluable information on how to feed them safely. The team may ask the parents/guardians to come to the school during mealtime and demonstrate how they feed the child at home. If the feeding techniques do not meet the recommendations that the team has made for the child then the team members need to share with the parents/guardians the evaluation and observations that resulted in the swallowing and feeding plan. In most cases parents appreciate the added information and welcome the effort to provide their child with a safe and efficient swallowing and feeding plan.

Knowing that the school team has looked at their child's history, has observed him or her, and has used an interdisciplinary team to determine how to meet the student's needs helps to relieve some of the stress related to raising a child with a swallowing and feeding disorder.

During the process of working with the student, the school team can ask parents what they feel would be helpful to them. The school district has many resources and can investigate caregivers, Medicaid programs, respite care, and other services. If the school district has social workers available to work with students and parents, the school team can refer the parents/guardians to them for help. School district teams can connect parents/guardians to support groups for families with children with disabilities. These services help families to address some of the concerns that have been mentioned and may help to reduce stress and anxiety (Box 8–2).

Cultural Considerations

A family's cultural values should be considered when writing a swallowing and feeding plan. In many cultures there are strong beliefs about which foods can or cannot be eaten, how foods are cooked or prepared, and how they are presented. The swallowing and feeding team needs to know and understand the family's cultural mores and learn about their beliefs about health, illness, and disorders and how they can impact what the swallowing and feeding team is able to do. Families with strong cultural beliefs about food may be very stressed and upset if their cultural customs are not considered. This may affect the relationship between the district and the family. When necessary, the district needs to have an interpreter available to help with determining the cultural values of the family (Davis-McFarland, 2008).

Long-Term, Proactive Commitment

Having a district-wide swallowing and feeding team procedure in place helps the swallowing and feeding team ensure that the

Box 8–2. Parent Perspective #2

Parent of a 4th-Grade Student With Mobius Syndrome and Significant Swallowing and Feeding Concerns

During an interview on her experience with the swallowing and feeding team at her child's school, the parent shared these thoughts on how the district helped her and her child:

Interviewer: How did the swallowing and feeding team help with your child's transition to school?

Mother: We were in the process of moving. The first district we went to said that because of her significant swallowing and feeding issues that they would not feed her at all at school. So we decided to look at the next district and they said that they had a dysphagia team and that they wanted her to come to their school. From the very beginning they just were real assertive with her issues and it made a world of difference in her speech, which helped her confidence and her safety in eating. We just saw her improve because she was getting therapy consistently at school. We really saw her confidence improve; she would hardly talk at all at school. I was a parent that I wanted everything to be about therapy. I was, let's take the bull by the horns here, I didn't want her to have any issues. I wanted it to be taken care of quickly. And the team said that we need to be sure that we approach this in a way that she's going to enjoy it and that she understands that eating is pleasurable. So I said all right. They helped me too, to try to make this fun for her. Which, I think, has helped her to be so cooperative in the long run because they started with such a good attitude and they helped her to have fun and they did some special things with her along the way.

Interviewer: What advice would you give therapists addressing swallowing and feeding in the schools?

Mother: The lady (SLP) that we worked with was just a wonderful example in that she made it fun for my daughter and she never, um, sometimes I would get frustrated and they were always so diplomatic and very professional. I really needed that because sometimes moms, they just, it's hard; it's really tough, because you want to see your child accepted and normal. So I really appreciated how they overlooked me sometimes when I would get impatient, you know, or frustrated, so that helped our relationship.

team has a system established to work closely with the parents/guardians. The second step of the procedure, after referral, is the parent interview. How the team approaches the parents/guardians from the very beginning shapes the relationship. Parents/guardians should be approached with respect and consideration. It is beneficial that from the first contact with the parents/guardians the school team provides the following:

- Description of the swallowing and feeding team. Identify who the school-based members of the team are and what their roles are in addressing the student's swallowing and feeding concerns. The role of the parents/guardians should also be discussed and feedback from the parents/guardians should be considered. They should be encouraged to be part of the problem-solving team, bringing with them their expertise on their child to share with the team.
- Information on the goals of the swallowing and feeding team at school
- Information on how the team will communicate with the parent to ensure that they always have current information on how their child is doing during mealtimes at schools (see Box 8–3)

Working With Parents/Guardians on Carryover of Swallowing and Feeding Skills to the Home Setting

Professionals in the schools work together to establish safe and efficient feeding that allows the child to participate, to the extent

Box 8–3. Parent Perspective #3

Mother of Two Children With Hunter Syndrome, a Rare Syndrome That Affects all Areas of Growth and Development Including Swallowing.

Children with this syndrome have a life expectancy of 12 to 18 years. During the interview on her experience with the swallowing and feeding team at her child's school, the parent shared these thoughts:

Mother: When the team came in they were really looking at a list of foods that are easy to choke on and they started saying: "He can't have this, he can't have this" and those happen to be foods that we packed every day. It seemed like we had all sticky foods, but when peanut butter was on bread, he was able to eat it, especially with jelly or honey. So initially I was not very happy because I felt that they didn't want me to send my child to school and eat at school. They were taking away the foods he did eat. From my standpoint I knew where the boys were going to be eventually and I didn't dwell on that, and I just looked at what they could do at the time. And so, I got a little defensive.

Interviewer: What could we have done better?

Mother: It got better. Everyone realized that my child was different than other children and that my two boys were different from each other. I think we all learned through the process. I learned to respect that the team could really help me and us as a family and the people that work with the boys and they learned from the boys because their syndrome is very rare and unique. Together we have worked and helped each other.

Interview: What advice would you like to give to therapists who are working with children with swallowing and feeding disorders?

> *Mother:* People have always said this but the parents truly do know their children better than anyone else. I think listen to the parents, first and foremost, and I think maybe having a session where they question the parents first and then come back. Instead of starting with what foods are typically bad for swallowing.
>
> *Interviewer:* Was there anything else you would like to say?
>
> *Mother:* I thank you for what you do; I think it is very important.

possible, with peers and family during mealtimes. When parents/guardians are involved throughout the process, the student progresses more quickly and there is often carryover to the home setting. As a result, one of the side benefits to establishing safe eating and progressing a student's diet at school is the potential to make a difference in the child's mealtimes at home.

Summary

This chapter has addressed some of the issues and concerns that parents/guardians of children with disabilities face. It has stressed the importance of trying to understand these issues and concerns and offered some suggestions for helping families. Handleman (1995, p. 361) stresses that "helping parents understand their child's disability, assisting them in coping with their feelings, and helping them make plans for their child's intervention are the challenges that face the professional." The school team clearly can have a positive effect on helping parents/guardians to adapt to their situation by working closely with them in a kind, understanding, and professional manner. Awareness of the challenges parents/guardians of children with disabilities face will help the school team to be emphatic and to offer support and assistance as the child goes through school.

Summary Sheet 4: Swallowing and Feeding in the Schools: Working With Parents/Guardians

Parents/Guardians Members of the Swallowing and Feeding Team!

- Explain district's swallowing and feeding team procedure when the student first enters the district.
- Discuss with the parents/guardians the district's goals for the student's swallowing and feeding at school.
- Encourage parents/guardians to share their knowledge of their child's feeding habits, food preferences, and mealtime environment.
- Interview parents/guardians to get medical information and history.
- Discuss with the parents/guardians the family's cultural views regarding food and mealtimes.
- Train parents to implement the swallowing and feeding plan at school and to reinforce oral/sensory therapy at home.

Understanding the Challenges Families Face

School district professionals should understand that:

- Feeding can be an emotional issue for parents/guardians.
- Families have many issues and concerns beyond school such as: medical, financial, and emotional issues.
- Parents/guardians may have fears in regard to the district swallowing and feeding team. For example, fear that the team will recommend non-oral feeding.
- Information shared with parents should be presented in lay terms with an effort to avoid alarming or scaring families.

continues

How Can a District Swallowing and Feeding Team Help the Parents/Guardians?

- Educate parents on the child's swallowing and feeding disorder, the signs and symptoms, and what they can do to help.
- Invest time in open and ongoing communication with parents/guardians in the form of notebooks, e-mails, phone calls, and conferences.
- Listen to what the parents/guardians have to say and seek their input in how they feed their child at home, including a demonstration at school.
- Connect the parents/guardians with other families and organizations that can offer support, guidance, and help.
- Follow the district procedure, which involves working closely with parents/guardians as members of the swallowing and feeding problem-solving team to foster a long-term, proactive commitment to the student's swallowing and feeding concerns.

References

Angell, M., Bailey, R., Nicholson, J., & Stoner, J. (2009). Family involvement in school-based dysphagia management. *Physical Disabilities: Education and Related Services, 28*(1), 6–24.

Brown, N. L., & Bhavnagri, N. (1996). *Effects of an early intervention program on stress and teaching ability of single mothers of young multiply impaired children.* U.S. Department of Education, Office of Educational Research and Improvement, Educational Resources Information Center. (ERIC Document Reproduction Service No. 398678), Michigan.

Davis-McFarland, E. (2008). Family and cultural issues in a school swallowing and feeding program. *Language, Speech, and Hearing Services in Schools, 39*(2), 199–213.

Gallagher, S., Phillips, A. C, Oliver, C., & Carroll, D. (2008). Predictors of psychological morbidity in parents of children with intellectual disability. *Journal of Pediatric Psychology, 33,* 1129–1136.

Garro, A., Thurman, S., Kerwin, M., & Ducette, J. (2005). Parent/Caregiver stress during pediatric hospitalization for chronic feeding problems. *Journal of Pediatric Nursing. 20*(4), 268–275.

Handleman, J. (1995). Raising a child with developmental disability: Understanding the family perspective. In S. Rosenthal, J. Sheppard, & M. Lotze (Eds.), *Dysphagia and the child with developmental disabilities* (pp. 355–361). San Diego, CA: Singular.

Homer, E. (2008). Establishing a public school dysphagia program. *Language, Speech, and Hearing Services in Schools, 39*(2), 177–187.

Horn, J. D., Feldman, H. M., & Ploof, D. L. (1995). Parent and professional perceptions about stress during a child's lengthy hospitalization. *Social Work in Health Care, 21,* 1107–1127.

Lopez, V., Clifford, T., Minnes, P., & Ouellette-Kuntz, H. (2008). Parental stress and coping in families of children with and without developmental delays. *Journal on Developmental Disabilities, 14*(2), 99–104.

9

Providing Swallowing and Feeding Services in the Schools: Training and Competency Issues

Emily M. Homer

Training and Competency

SLPs working in school districts have advance knowledge in articulation, fluency, voice, and language disorders in school-aged children. They often know and understand the importance of language in emerging literacy and are able to address language-based academic weaknesses in their students. These are specialty areas that school-based SLPs have spent years developing and it is something they are very comfortable addressing. The same can be said for hospital-based SLP's expertise in the areas of swallowing and feeding with the adult population. School-based SLPs, however, do not often work on or have much experience with swallowing and feeding disorders and in many cases have not developed those skills. As a district adopts a swallowing and feeding procedure it is essential that district administrators are aware of the training gaps that may exist and be willing to provide a path for school-based SLPs to update and develop the knowledge and skills that they will need to manage swallowing and feeding disorders in the schools. It is also important for OTs and nurses to acquire the skills they need to address swallowing and feeding in the school setting. This chapter offers some solutions to training and competency issues in districts addressing swallowing and feeding.

District Responsibility

It is important for a school district to support professionals working with students by ensuring that they are well trained and are able to teach their subject matter. In the area of swallowing and feeding this takes on a different level of importance. When a speech-language pathologist is inadequately prepared to treat a child with an articulation disorder, it is serious because that child may not progress or may not perform as well in class or socially. However, in the case of swallowing and feeding, the inadequate training and preparation of a treating therapist can result in a medical situation such as choking, aspiration, and/or very serious illness (Power-deFur, 2000). There continues to be many students in school districts throughout the country who are being fed by well-intentioned classroom teachers in a manner that not only does not meet the nutritional requirements of the student, but also puts them at significant health risks. Although SLPs, OTs, and nurses working in the schools typically do not have the intense experience working with swallowing and feeding that their colleagues in other settings have; they often have the basic skills that they learned in school, which can then be supplemented with additional training and experience. The knowledge and skills they bring from their training programs allow them to be able to work to establish safe eating at school for students with swallowing and feeding disorders. One of the worst situations for children with swallowing and feeding disorders is for the school system to do nothing. By ignoring the concerns, the district is allowing the child to be fed in a manner that may compromise their health and is putting their professional staff in a situation where they have an ethical dilemma.

There is always the option of outside referral or for the district to contract with trained professionals.

A study by O'Donoghue and Dean-Claytor (2008) looked at the training of school-based SLPs and their reported confidence in treating children with swallowing and feeding disorders. The results found that therapists who participated in continuing education in the area of swallowing and feeding, within 2 years of the study, reported higher confidence ratings than those who had not participated recently in specific professional development. This suggests that by making professional development opportunities available to therapists, not only does the therapist improve his or her knowledge but they also become more confident in treating children with the disorder.

A district that establishes a swallowing and feeding team procedure will need to support their personnel by providing additional training, collaboration time, and mentoring in the area of swallowing and feeding. Having well-trained professionals in the school setting is an achievable goal and one that a district should support.

Importance of Professional Competency and the Code of Ethics

All professionals have a responsibility to be competent in the area they are working and to maintain that competency. Every SLP, OT, and registered nurse is obligated to follow the requirements laid out in their Code of Ethics. Although all areas of the Code of Ethics are important, and in many ways apply to school-based swallowing and feeding services, there are two areas that are particularly relevant and warrant mentioning.

Competency: Obtaining and Maintaining

There are specific knowledge and skills that the core team members, the SLP, OT, and nurse, must have in order to work with children with swallowing and feeding disorders. The national organizations for each of the three professions have language in their Code of Ethics that stresses the importance and responsibility of acquiring the knowledge and skills needed to effectively work with a disorder. Following are quotes from each organization:

According to the American Speech-Language-Hearing Association Code of Ethics (ASHA, 2010), "individuals shall engage in only those aspects of the professions that are within the scope of their professional practice and competence, considering their level of education, training, and experience. In addition, SLPs have a responsibility to "maintain and enhance professional competence and performance."

Under the American Occupational Therapy Association Code of Ethics (AOTA, 2010), Beneficence, Principle 1, occupational therapy personnel shall demonstrate a concern for the well-being and safety of the recipients of their services by taking responsible steps (e.g., continuing education, research, supervision, training) and use careful judgment to ensure their own competence and weigh potential for client harm when generally recognized standards do not exist in emerging technology or areas of practice.

In similar language to the SLP and OT Code of Ethics, the American Nurses Association (ANA), states "the nurse owes the same duties to self as to others, including the responsibility to preserve integrity and safety, to maintain competence, and to continue personal and professional growth."

Professionals working in school systems have the same professional requirements to follow their association's Code of Ethics as those working in other settings. Many who work in school districts have never been responsible for diagnosing and treating children with swallowing and feeding disorders and therefore may not have the knowledge and skills to work with them. They cannot go against their Code of Ethics and, as a result, are responsible for obtaining and maintaining competency so that they can address the child's swallowing and feeding issues.

Competency: Safety of Client/Patient

All three professions stress the importance of providing high-quality, effective services to their clients/patients. According to each discipline's Code of Ethics the services provided must benefit the client/patient and cannot harm them.

ASHA's Code of Ethics (2010) states, "individuals shall honor their responsibility to hold paramount the welfare of persons they serve professionally."

Language within the AOTA (2010) states specifically that the OT has "an obligation to not impose risks of harm even if the potential risk is without malicious or harmful intent."

The Code of Ethics for nurses' states, "the nurse promotes, advocates for, and strives to protect the health, safety, and rights of the patient." The nurse is responsible primarily to the patient and their health and safety. "Nurses are accountable for judgments made and actions taken in the course of nursing practice, irrespective of healthcare organizations' policies or providers' directives (ANA, 2015)."

The issue of health and safety will come up when diagnosing and treating children with swallowing and feeding disorders in the school setting. Each student with a health and safety issue needs to be considered separately based on the information available. The professionals trained in swallowing and feeding disorders evaluate the situation and determine if there are ways that the student can eat safely and efficiently at school. School districts already have the responsibility to ensure that students are safe at school and each professional has an ethical responsibility to make sure that the treatments they are providing are safe and do not harm children. For example, when a trained professional, such as an SLP, observes that a child is unable to chew the food that is prepared for him or her, then they have an obligation to that child to refer the child to the swallowing and feeding team (see Appendix A). The team needs to determine the extent of the child's difficulty eating and establish a swallowing and feeding plan (see Appendix B) that provides a means for the child to eat safely. It is the ethical responsibility for those professionals to alter the child's feeding to ensure his or her safety. This should be done immediately while the team is in the process of working with the parents and doing a thorough evaluation of the child's swallowing and feeding skills. The trained professional cannot allow the child to be fed at school in a manner that compromises the student's health. In the example, the school team would write a temporary Swallowing and Feeding Plan (see Appendix B) that would include finely chopped foods and would restrict the child's meals to items that could be finely chopped or that were a smooth texture and did not require much chewing. The plan may also include a controlled bite size and slower rate of intake. This plan would establish safer feeding at school until the entire procedure was completed and the team had all the necessary information to establish a plan. During this process, the importance of working with the parents is stressed.

Determining Professional Competency in a School District

It is the responsibility of each school district to ensure that the professionals who work for them have the certification, knowledge, and skills to work in their area. Many school-based SLPs, OTs, and nurses may have little or no training and experience in swallowing and feeding disorders. As a district establishes an interdisciplinary swallowing and feeding team, it will need to determine the level of training and experience in swallowing and feeding disorders that each relevant staff member has in order for them to be able to address the complex issues that may occur in the district when addressing this disorder.

Survey of District Personnel

Once a district has made the decision to establish a swallowing and feeding team and put into place a swallowing and feeding procedure, one of the first steps will be to determine the number of trained professionals they have on staff. Almost all school districts employ SLPs, OTs, and nurses in some capacity.

Speech-Language Pathologists

SLPs who have received their Masters level degree in the past 15 years have had coursework and practicum in swallowing (dysphagia) and feeding with an emphasis on dysphagia. OT programs address feeding, eating, and swallowing in their program, with an emphasis on feeding and eating. Nursing programs cover the anatomy and physiology of the swallowing and feeding mechanism but typically do not offer or require a course or practicum in swallowing disorders. In most districts the SLP will be the professional with the most knowledge, skills, training, and experience in swallowing and feeding; however, it is possible that SLPs employed in the schools have either never been trained or have been trained but have never used their skills. It will be important for a school district to determine the SLPs in the district who are trained, experienced, and able to take a leadership role in updating the skills of other SLPs in the district.

The designated swallowing and feeding team administrator can send out a survey of the following to all district employed SLPs:

- Have you had a graduate level course in dysphagia?
- Have you had clinical practicum experience in graduate school in the area of dysphagia or feeding disorders? If so, approximately, how many hours of practicum do you have and what was the location(s) (e.g., hospital, skilled nursing facility, etc.)?
- Have you ever worked in a hospital, skilled nursing facility, home health, and so forth where dysphagia was a large percentage of your workload? If yes, for how long?
- Have you attended any continuing education courses or sessions on any of the following: dysphagia, feeding disorders, swallowing and feeding in the schools, pediatric dysphagia, and so forth?

Occupational Therapists

Many OTs have worked in hospital settings prior to coming to the schools and may have specific experience in swallowing and feeding. They also typically have coursework that addresses feeding, eating, and swallowing according to their national organization, AOTA. It will be helpful for a district to survey their OTs to determine which ones are most qualified to serve as leaders in the area of swallowing and feeding. The designated swallowing and feeding team administrator can send out a survey of the following to all district employed OTs:

- Please rate your knowledge and skills in the area of swallowing and feeding, according to the Specialized Knowledge and Skills in Feeding, Eating, and Swallowing for Occupational Therapy Practice: (a) entry level knowledge and skills, (b) advanced level knowledge and skills.

- Have you had fieldwork experience in graduate school in feeding, eating, and/or swallowing disorders? If so, approximately, how many hours of fieldwork do you have and what was the location(s) (e.g., hospital, skilled nursing facility, etc.)?
- Have you ever worked in a hospital where you addressed swallowing and feeding disorders? If yes, where was it and what was your role?
- Have you attended any continuing education courses or sessions on any of the following: dysphagia, feeding disorders, swallowing and feeding in the schools, pediatric dysphagia, and so forth?

School Nurses

Nurses are trained extensively on all of the health issues and concerns that arise when a patient has dysphagia or a behavioral feeding disorders. They know the signs and symptoms of under-nutrition and dehydration, aspiration, gastro esophageal reflux, seizures, and so forth. They may not be trained in dysphagia specifically and will rely on the SLP to train them on the particulars of recognizing a swallowing disorder and the risks that can occur. District employed nurses will have the basic information needed for them to be active, effective team members. They will benefit from additional training and professional development in swallowing and feeding disorders and their role.

Self-Review of School-Based Personnel Using Knowledge and Skills Documents

There is language in both ASHA and AOTA organizations that professionals in both fields are responsible for ensuring that they have the training to work with the populations under their care. Both of these organizations publish Knowledge and Skills documents to assist professionals in determining the level of their skills and the areas where additional knowledge is indicated.

Knowledge and Skills Needed by Speech-Language Pathologists Providing Services to Individuals With Swallowing and/or Feeding Disorders

The American Speech-Language-Hearing Association knowledge and skills document (ASHA, 2002) gives the SLP a tool that outlines the basic competencies necessary for the SLP wanting to address swallowing and feeding disorders. These "basic competencies" are part of a graduate level course that is required by ASHA to include swallowing (oral, pharyngeal, esophageal, and related functions, including oral function for feeding, orofacial myology). In addition, all SLPs currently in a graduate level program have clinical practicum in the area of swallowing and feeding. The knowledge and skills document provides the practicing SLP with the specific skills that are needed for the setting they are working so every speech-language pathologist will not necessarily need to develop proficiencies in all roles. In a clinical role the SLP will need to develop proficiencies based on the populations served (e.g., adult, head and neck cancer, pediatrics), but the SLP in an administrative role would require extensive experience in supervision. It is recommended that achievement of proficiencies be documented and that the school-based professional systematically plan a process for attaining proficiency for serving individuals with swallowing and feeding problems in the school setting.

For example, the SLP working in the school setting would need to have a basic understanding of the modified barium swallow study and to know what they are observing when they attend a study; however, they would not be required to conduct the study, analyze it, or write the report. Those would not be knowledge and skills that they would need in their role as a school-based SLP.

Specialized Knowledge and Skills in Feeding, Eating, and Swallowing for Occupational Therapy

The Specialized Knowledge and Skills in Feeding, Eating, and Swallowing for Occupational Therapy (2007) provides the practicing OT with a document that outlines the skills needed to address feeding, eating, and swallowing at the entry level and also at the advanced level. OTs with Masters degrees have the entry level skills outlined in this document. The progression from entry level knowledge and skills to advanced-level knowledge and skills is individualized and could be obtained by maintaining and documenting competence in practice, education, and research and by participating in professional development, educational activities, and critical examination of available evidence (AOTA, 2007). The OT professional has the responsibility to ensure that they are competent in the services they provide, including swallowing and feeding services. The document can be used by school-based OTs to self-review their knowledge and skills and to seek out professional development and training in the areas that they do not feel competent.

District Plan for Establishing and Maintaining Professional Competency in the Area of Swallowing and Feeding

Although diagnosing and treating swallowing and feeding involves a team process, in most districts it is the SLP who will have the most training and as a result will be responsible for managing the cases. Both the school nurse and the OT have the basic skills to support and address specific areas of the disorder; however, it is the SLP who has the training and skills in all phases of swallowing. Once a district has surveyed their personnel and knows how many SLPs they employ who have the knowledge and skills to address swallowing and feeding disorders in children then they will need to establish a plan for working with them to establish and to maintain competency.

The District With No Trained SLPs or Only SLPs Who Have Never Used Their Skills

It is possible that a school district may only employ SLPs who have never had coursework or training in dysphagia or who were trained a long time ago and have never used their skills. In those cases, there are some options that districts can utilize to be able to begin working with students with swallowing and feeding disorders. If the district has no SLPs who are competent to diagnose and treat children with dysphagia they can:

- Hire an SLP with the necessary knowledge, skills, and experience to work with the students who have the disorder and can work on training other therapists to assist.
- Contract with a health care agency to provide SLPs who have training and experience in swallowing and feeding, to set up swallowing and feeding plans, and to work with the students and the school staff.
- Partner with a local university to offer a graduate level swallowing and feeding course, after school hours, that is available to school-based SLPs to begin the process of updating their skills. The district can also work with the university to offer the course for the district SLPs where the district would sponsor the course.
- If the SLPs have had a course but have not used the skills, then the district can provide opportunities for them to attend professional development. The district can sponsor speakers who can provide training or can allow release time and stipends for SLPs to attend conferences, conventions, presentations, and so forth.

Updating the Knowledge and Skills of SLPs Who Have Some Competency in Swallowing and Feeding

It is more likely that a school district will have some SLPs who have graduate level coursework, practicum and some experience in diagnosing and treating swallowing and feeding. For these therapists and other core team members it will be necessary for the school district to offer opportunities to update their skills and to provide ongoing professional development specific to working with children from 3 to 22 years old.

The amount and type of professional development will depend on the district itself. Some small districts will find it more cost effective to send their core team members, SLPs, OTs, and nurses, to professional development offered in nearby communities. All three professions have organizations that have state and national conventions. In addition, there are many private companies that offer courses in larger communities that focus on specific areas. For example, the SLPs can attend sessions that focus on pharyngeal and esophageal phase dysphagia, while OTs can attend sessions that focus on positioning or sensory feeding issues. Nurses can seek out sessions that address pharmacology and respiratory compromise as a result of aspiration in special populations.

Some school districts may have the means to bring in national speakers on swallowing and feeding to train their personnel. This is an effective way to get many therapists and nurses trained at one time. Then the district can follow up training by having therapists within their district prepare presentations on specific issues and specific types of cases. This type of training can then be customized to meet the needs of the swallowing and feeding team in the district. The district can pay to have university professors and hospital SLPs come and provide additional training.

There are many high-quality webinar and recorded sessions that can be viewed as a group or can be purchased by the school district. These trainings are often reasonable and can fill in some of the training gaps within the district. Allowing the core team members training time to get together and view these would be an effective way to continually update skills. Shared learning occurs when a group views the same sessions and stop to periodically have a discussion on the content. This is an extremely effective way to learn new information and to augment the knowledge already obtained.

Ongoing Professional Development

Once the district's team is established and they are implementing the swallowing and feeding team procedure, ongoing professional development will be necessary for employees to continuously update and maintain skills. The district should take the responsibility for providing opportunities for the SLPs, OTs, and nurses to receive high-quality professional development yearly on swallowing and feeding disorders. There are many options today for professional development and shared learning. These include:

- University sponsored sessions
- Professional organizations sponsored conventions and sessions both state and national
- Hospital sponsored training
- Private continuing education company sponsored sessions
- School system sponsored sessions designed to meet the needs of district employees

Mentoring and Collaboration

In addition to professional development, it is recommended that professionals working with students with swallowing and feeding disorders have opportunities to meet and discuss cases with one another. Swallowing and feeding in the school setting is a low-incidence disorder. Most SLPs, OTs, and nurses, depending on the model chosen by the district, will only have a few students a year to follow and treat for swallowing and feeding. They would benefit from meeting with other case managers to discuss cases and problem solve. This would result in expanding their experience and knowledge base.

Some therapists will have a lot of experience with swallowing and feeding in a different setting. These therapists can serve as leaders and mentors to those who have training but limited experience. These therapists can help initially with decision making and problem solving. In some cases, the district may invite hospital SLPs or university SLPs to come help school therapists to hone their skills while getting support from a therapist with more experience. In most districts there will be a way to improve the competency of the school therapy staff and begin to serve children with swallowing and feeding disorders.

Individual Learning

SLPs, OTs, or nurses have opportunities to learn on their own. There are many sources for acquiring information and each professional will be able to design their training to meet their own individual needs. The knowledge and skills documents can serve as a guide for the SLP and OT to determine where their weak areas are and to seek out additional information. Learning may consist of reading current research in the area, attending lectures and presentations, viewing webinars and recorded sessions, observing SLPs or OTs working in the area, researching and preparing a presentation to share with others, as well as many other means of professional growth. The opportunities for learning and updating skills are almost limitless for the motivated professional.

Swallowing and Feeding Team Administrator

The school district's swallowing and feeding team administrator should be knowledgeable and trained in the identification and treatment of swallowing and feeding disorders. The administrator should have the experience, skills, and time to serve as a consultant and mentor other therapists in the district. In many cases, when there are concerns, the swallowing and feeding team administrator should be available to discuss cases with team members, and attend IEP meetings and instrumental swallow studies. The team administrator needs training in the legal aspects of identifying and treating swallowing and feeding disorders and serves as a support to team members when legal issues come up.

Summary of Training and Competency

All professionals have the responsibility to acquire and maintain competency in the areas that they work. In many cases, SLPs, OTs, and nurses working in the school setting will need to obtain, update, or maintain training specific to addressing swallowing and feeding disorders in the school setting. The district should work with their personnel to offer opportunities, funds, and release time to acquire the necessary training to work with this population. It can be done in many ways, using many sources. This combination of the individual professional taking responsibility for their own competency and the district supporting and encouraging training will result in a staff that is able to address the complex issues around identifying and treating a child with a swallowing and feeding disorder using a team approach.

References

American Nurses Association. (2015). *Code of ethics for nurses.* Retrieved from http://www.nursingworld.org/MainMenuCategories/Ethics Standards/CodeofEthicsforNurses

American Occupational Therapy Association. (2007). Specialized knowledge and skills in feeding, eating, and swallowing for occupational therapy. *American Journal of Occupational Therapy, 61*(November/December), 686–700.

American Occupational Therapy Association. (2010). AOTA official document in AJOT online supplement. *American Journal of Occupational Therapy, 64*(November/December Suppl.), 827.

American Speech-Language-Hearing Association. (2002). *Knowledge and skills needed by speech-language pathologists providing services to individuals with swallowing and/or feeding disorders* [Knowledge and skills]. Retrieved from http://www.asha.org/policy

American Speech-Language-Hearing Association. (2010). *Code of ethics* [Ethics]. Retrieved from http://www.asha.org/policy

O'Donoghue, C., & Dean-Claytor, A. (2008). Training and self-reported confidence for dysphagia management among speech-language pathologists in the schools. *Language, Speech, and Hearing Services in Schools, 39,* 192–197.

Power-deFur, L. (2000). Serving students wit dysphagia in the schools? Educational preparation is essential! *Language, Speech, and Hearing Services in Schools, 31,* 76–78.

APPENDIX A

Swallowing and Feeding Team Referral Form

School District Name: _____

Date Form Completed: _____

Student: _____

Date of Birth: _____

School: _____

Classroom Teacher: _____

Completed By/Title: _____

Please check all that apply:

Medical Information
☐ Repeated respiratory infections
☐ Vocal cord paralysis
☐ Medical HX of swallowing problems
☐ History of head injury
☐ History of recurring pneumonia
☐ Cleft palate
☐ HX of GERD
☐ Weight loss/failure to thrive

Observed Behaviors
☐ Requires special diet or diet modification (i.e. baby foods, thickener, soft food only)
☐ Poor upper body control
☐ Poor oral motor functioning
☐ Maintains open mouth posture
☐ Drooling

- [ ] Nasal regurgitation
- [ ] Food remains in mouth after meals (pocketing)
- [ ] Wet breath sounds and/or gurgly voice quality following meals or drinking
- [ ] Coughing/choking during meals
- [ ] Swallowing solid food without chewing
- [ ] Effortful swallowing
- [ ] Eyes watering/tearing during mealtime
- [ ] Unusual head/neck posturing during eating
- [ ] Hypersensitive gag reflex
- [ ] Food and/or drink escaping from the mouth or trach tube
- [ ] Slurred speech
- [ ] Mealtime takes more than 30 minutes
- [ ] Overstuffing

Additional Reported or Observed Behaviors
- [ ] Feeding aversion
- [ ] Feeding jags (eats only one thing)
- [ ] Limited eating (only eats a certain amount)
- [ ] Food refusal
- [ ] Spitting up or vomiting associated with eating and drinking

Additional information or comments: _____

_____

_____

Note. Printed with permission from the St. Tammany Parish Schools Special Education Department (2015).

APPENDIX B
Swallowing and Feeding Plan Form

School District Name: _____

Date of Plan: _____

Review Date: _____

Student: _____

Date of Birth: _____

School: _____

Teacher: _____

Dysphagia Case Manager: _____

If there are any questions regarding this student's feeding plan, please contact the Case Manager at the following:

Location(s): _____

Phone #s: _____ _____

Case History: _____

_____

Feeding Recommendations:

Positioning: _____

Equipment: _____

Tube Fed: ☐ tube fed/nothing by mouth ☐ tube and oral fed

(amount fed orally: _____)

Diet/Food Prep:

Food Consistency: ☐ Pureed ☐ Ground ☐ Chopped

☐ Mashed ☐ Bite-sized

Liquid Consistency: ☐ No liquids ☐ Thin liquids

☐ Thickened liquids (circle)

nector honey pudding

Other: _____

Feeding Plan Techniques/Precautions:

Amount of food per bite: _____

Food placement: _____

☐ Keep student in upright position _____ minutes after meal.

☐ Offer a drink after _____ bites.

Additional precautions/comments:

_____

_____

Feeding/Swallowing Plan In Service Training:

I, the undersigned, have read and been trained on implementing
the feeding/swallowing plan for _____.
I agree to follow the swallowing plan as specified.

Name	Position	Date Review	Date
_____	_____	_____	_____
_____	_____	_____	_____
_____	_____	_____	_____
_____	_____	_____	_____

I understand that I am responsible for the implementation of
the swallowing and feeding plan in my classroom.

Signed: _____ (classroom teacher)

Date: _____

Note. Printed with permission from the St. Tammany Parish Schools
Special Education Department (2015).

APPENDIX C

Swallowing and Feeding Team Case Manager Transfer Form

School District Name: _____

Please complete this form on any student who will be moving or has moved to a new school. Put a copy of this form in the student's folder and send a copy of this transfer form to the swallowing and feeding administrator. Complete a different form for each student who is transferring to a different school.

Date: _____

Name of Student: _____

Date of Birth: _____

Current School: _____

Current Case Manager: _____

School Transferring to: _____

Receiving Case Manager: _____

Note. Printed with permission from the St. Tammany Parish Schools Special Education Department (2015).

APPENDIX D
Parental/Guardian Interview Form

School District Name: _____
☐ Meeting
☐ Phone

Student: _____

Sex: _____

Date of Birth: _____

Name of Parents: _____

Phone: _____

Address: _____

Do you have any concerns about your child's feeding and/or mealtimes? ☐ YES ☐ NO

If yes, please describe: _____

Medical Information

Name of primary care physician: _____

Is your child followed by any of the following physicians?

☐ Gastroenterologist
  Name & Phone #: _____

☐ Neurologist
  Name & Phone #: _____

☐ Pulmonologist
  Name & Phone #: _____

Current Height: _____

Current Weight: _____

Allergies, including food allergies: _____

_____

Bowel Habits:

Frequency of Bowel Movements: _____ times per
(check one): □ Day □ Week

Consistency: □ Hard □ Soft □ Loose □ Watery

Medications taken on a regular basis (please include dosage
and frequency):

Medication	Dose	Prescribing Physician

Please check if your child has had the test below:

□ Swallow study (MBSS/VFSS)

Date: _____ Results: _____

□ Upper GI (Barium Study)

Date: _____ Results: _____

□ Gastric emptying

Date: _____ Results: _____

Does or has your child ever had GERD (gastroesphogeal reflux
disorder)? If yes, please list the symptoms and treatments:

_____

_____

Has your child ever been diagnosed failure to thrive?

□ YES/when?: _____ □ No

Explain how this was addressed:

_____

_____

Was it resolved? _____

Was or is your child fed through a feeding tube?   □ YES   □ NO

If yes, then when? How long? _____

What was the reason for the tube feeding?

□ Aspiration   □ Failure to thrive   □ Other: _____

Hospitalizations (month, year, reason): _____

_____

Current medical problems:

_____

_____

Dental Information

Does your child visit the dentist on a regular basis?
□ YES   □ NO

When was your child's last visit to the dentist?

Date: _____   Dentist: _____

Is there any significant dental history that may affect your child's eating habits?   □ YES   □ NO

If yes, please explain:

_____

_____

Tooth brushing: □ with assistance   □ independent

Current Feeding Practices

Describe a typical family meal:

_____

_____

What are your child's food preferences?

Likes	Dislikes
_____	_____
_____	_____
_____	_____

What kinds of food does your child eat?

☐ Regular liquids   ☐ Thickened liquids   ☐ Pureed
☐ Mashed   ☐ Ground   ☐ Chopped   ☐ Bite-sized pieces
☐ Table foods (whatever your family is eating)

Does your child feed himself/herself?

☐ YES, independently   ☐ YES, with assistance   ☐ NO

Does your child enjoy mealtime?

_____

How do you know when your child is hungry?

_____

How do you know when your child is full?

_____

Frequency and duration of meals:

_____

Check all that apply:

- ☐ Choking during a meal
- ☐ Difficulty chewing
- ☐ Coughing with or without spraying of food
- ☐ Chronic respiratory problems (pneumonia)
- ☐ Chronic ear infections
- ☐ Tongue thrust
- ☐ Gurgly or "wet" voice
- ☐ Biting on utensils
- ☐ Vomiting
- ☐ Gagging
- ☐ Food refusal
- ☐ Sensitive to being touched around the mouth
- ☐ Drooling: ___ constant ___ frequent ___ occasional
- ☐ Avoidance behaviors during feeding

Does your child take any nutritional supplements?

☐ YES   ☐ NO   If yes, specify _____

Do certain foods/liquids appear to be more difficult for your child to eat?

_____

_____

How is your child positioned during feeding?

- ☐ Regular chair at table
- ☐ High chair
- ☐ Tumble form chair
- ☐ Adaptive chair, type: _____
- ☐ Other: _____
- ☐ Booster seat
- ☐ Sitting in a wheelchair
- ☐ Held on lap

What utensils are used?

- ☐ Bottle
- ☐ Sippy cup
- ☐ Cup (no lid)
- ☐ Straw
- ☐ Spoon
- ☐ Fork
- ☐ Toddler utensils

Other adaptive equipment _____

_____

Additional comments or concerns: _____

_____

_____

Parent Signature   **Date**

Parent's Name Printed   **Phone #**

Interviewed By   **Position**   **Date**

Note. Printed with permission from the St. Tammany Parish Schools
Special Education Department (2015).

APPENDIX E

Interdisciplinary Observation Form

School District Name: _____

Student: _____

Age: _____

Date of Birth: _____

Date of Observation: _____

School: _____

Exceptionality: _____

SLP: _____

OT: _____

Classroom Teacher: _____

Nurse: _____

Parent: _____

Observation of Foods Presented

Write in the name of the food presented in the blocks labeled food 1, food 2, and food 3. Below the name of the food, write the consistency of the food presented: pureed, ground, mashed, chopped, or bite size. Put + for yes observed or − for no not observed in each box to indicate whether a behavior was observed or not with that particular food and consistency.

Person administering food: _____

Location/setting: _____

Positioning: _____

	Food 1	Food 2	Food 3
Consistency of food presented			
Poor lip closure			
Drooling			
Reduced lip action to clear material			
Poor bolus formation/ movement			
Decreased anterior/posterior movement			
Food residue in oral cavity			
Absence of chewing			
Absence of rotary jaw movement (munching)			
Bites on spoon or utensil			
Delayed swallow initiation: ant/ post-swallow delay			
Cough or throat clear following swallow	_____ seconds	_____ seconds	_____ seconds
Cued swallow			
Fatigues easily			
Gagging before/ during/after meal			

Observation of Liquids Presented

Write in the name of the liquid presented in the blocks labeled liquid 1, liquid 2, and liquid 3. Below the name of the liquid, write the consistency of the liquid: unthickened, nectar, honey, or pudding. Put + for yes observed or − for no not observed in each box to indicate whether a behavior was observed or not with that particular liquid and consistency.

Method of presentation (e.g., straw, etc):

	Liquid 1	Liquid 2	Liquid 3
Consistency of liquid			
Tongue thrust/ reduced retraction			
Bite on cup			
Anterior loss			
Limited jaw opening			
Limited upper lip closure over cup			
Delayed swallow			
Coughing following drink			

Behavioral Observations

Briefly describe how the food was presented and what happened under each presentation. Put + if the behavior was observed and − if the behavior was not observed.

Interfering Behaviors	Presentation #1	Presentation #2	Presentation #3
Throwing food/ utensils + beh. obs. − beh. not obs.			
Screaming/crying + beh. obs. − beh. not obs.			
Self-injury + beh. obs. − beh. not obs.			
Flopping (falling to the floor) + beh. obs. − beh. not obs.			
Leaving the area + beh. obs. − beh. not obs.			
Closing mouth/ head turn + beh. obs. − beh. not obs.			
Talking with food in mouth + beh. obs. − beh. not obs.			
Spitting + beh. obs. − beh. not obs.			

Interfering Behaviors	Presentation #1	Presentation #2	Presentation #3
Overstuffing + beh. obs. − beh. not obs.			
Aggression (biting, scratching, head butting, punching, using objects to attempt to hurt the feeder) + beh. obs. − beh. not obs.			
Self-induced gagging/vomiting + beh. obs. − beh. not obs.			

Sensory Questionnaire and Observation

Observe and interview teachers, parents, and others and indicate if each statement applies. Add comments to explain further.

Sensory Questionnaire/ Observation	√ if statement applies	Additional comments:
Avoids eating certain food textures (crunchy, soft, chewy, liquid)		
Avoids eating foods of certain temperatures (warm like oatmeal, cold like ice, room temperature)		
Eats primarily one color of food		
Eats only certain tastes (salty, sweet, sour, spicy, bland)		
Does not notice food left on his or her face		
Reacts emotionally when asked to hold utensil/cup		
Limits self to specific food items (list food)		
Gags when introducing a new food or texture		
Gags easily when eating or when using utensils		
Resists tactile exploration of food or other activities (sand, mud, playdough, etc.)		

Sensory Questionnaire/ Observation	√ if statement applies	Additional comments:
Enjoys playing with food but does not eat it		
Resists grooming: face washing, tooth brushing		
Mouths, licks, or chews non-edible items		
Routinely smells things (food or non-food items)		
Sensitive to sounds (e.g., cafeteria)		

Modifications Attempted During Interdisciplinary Observation

Dietary modifications:

_____

Liquid modifications:

_____

Adapted equipment modifications:

_____

Positional changes:

_____

Behavioral interventions:

_____

Other:

_____

Summary and Findings

_____

_____

_____

_____

_____

_____

Recommendations

1. _____

_____

_____

_____

2. _____

_____

_____

_____

3. _____

_____

_____

_____

Referral for:

☐ MBSS

☐ GI

☐ Physician Consultation

☐ Physician Orders

☐ Behavioral Referral (CAAB)

☐ Swallowing and Feeding Plan

☐ Emergency Plan

☐ Training

Note. Printed with permission from the St. Tammany Parish Schools Special Education Department (2015).

APPENDIX F
Pre-lEP Conference Form

School District Name: _____

Student: _____

Date of Conference: _____

School: _____

Teacher: _____

Attendees Sign In

Name: _____ Discipline: _____

Name: _____ Discipline: _____

Name: _____ Discipline: _____

Name: _____ Discipline: _____

Name: _____ Discipline: _____

Name: _____ Discipline: _____

Issues Discussed/Recommendations

1. Liquid modifications: _____

_____

2. Dietary modifications: _____

_____

3. Sensory/motor observations: _____

_____

4. Behavioral modifications: _____

_____

5. Adaptive equipment modifications: _____

_____

6. Positional changes: _____

_____

Additional information or comments:

_____

_____

_____

_____

APPENDIX G
Prescription of School Meal Modification Form

Please return to the school. For the safety of the student, this form MUST be thoroughly and legibly completed.

School District Name: _____

Student's Name: _____

Age: _____

School: _____

Grade/Classroom: _____

Parent's Name: _____

Parent's E-mail: _____

Address: _____

Telephone: _____

List the medical condition that requires special nutritional or feeding needs:

_____

_____

Diet Prescription (mark all that apply)

Food Intolerance:

Eliminate ALL foods that may contain any form of:

☐ Eggs—pure form only   ☐ Eggs Proteins

☐ Milk-beverage form only*   ☐ Fish

   *Substitute (please circle) Juice or Water   ☐ Milk Proteins

☐ Milk AND Dairy only*   ☐ Nuts

   *Substitute (please circle) Juice or Water   ☐ Peanuts

☐ Soy—pure form only   ☐ Shellfish

☐ Wheat-whole or unprocessed only   ☐ Soy

☐ Other   ☐ Wheat

Consistency Only:

☐ Puree

☐ Mechanical Soft

☐ Chopped

Any Other Specific Dietary Need:

_____

*Please note if juice or water may be substituted for liquid milk. If juice or water substitute is not noted on diet prescription form, student will be charged for juice or water.

Specific Foods to Omit   Specific Foods to Substitute

_____   _____

_____   _____

_____   _____

I certify that the above named student needs special meals prepared as described above because of the student's chronic medical condition:

Office Address: _____

Office Telephone: _____

Office Fax: _____

_____   _____
Licensed Physician/Recognized   Date
Medical Authority Signature

Note. Printed with permission from the St. Tammany Parish Schools Special Education Department (2015).

APPENDIX H

Pre-Instrumental Examination Information Form

School District Name: _____

Date Form Completed: _____

Name: _____

Date of Birth: _____

Diagnosis: _____

C.A.: _____

Referring SLP: _____

Brief Medical History:

_____

_____

_____

Positional Concerns/Adaptive Equipment Currently Used at School:

_____

_____

Current Diet:

Home: _____

School: _____

Summary of Interdisciplinary Observation:

The following was observed during a clinical observation of the student's feeding and swallowing at school.

Oral Phase

☐ drooling

☐ pocketing   ☐ lateral sulcus   ☐ anterior sulcus

☐ not clearing the oral cavity before swallow

☐ anterior loss/poor lip seal

☐ excessive chewing

☐ hyper/hypo sensitivity

☐ difficulty with bolus formation

Pharyngeal Phase

☐ coughing/choking: ☐ before   ☐ after   ☐ during swallow

☐ delay in triggering swallow

☐ wet/gurgly voice quality after swallow

☐ decreased/absent laryngeal elevation

☐ expectorating food

☐ repetitive swallows

Information that the school system would like to get from the MBSS/VFSS/FEES is as follows:

1. _____

2. _____

3. _____

4. _____

Additional Comments/Concerns:

_____

We have included an Authorization for Release of Confidential Information.

Note. Printed with permission from the St. Tammany Parish Schools Special Education Department (2015).

APPENDIX I
Swallowing and Feeding Team Procedure Checklist

Student: _____

School: _____

SLP: _____

OT: _____

Nurse: _____

DATE   **PROCEDURE**

_____ Referral form completed and sent to Dysphagia Coordinator

_____ Parent interview completed

_____ Interdisciplinary observation conducted

　　　　　 _____ Preconference held (non-behavior feeding)

　　　　　 _____ Interim Swallowing and Feeding Plan established

　　　　　 _____ Interim Emergency Plan established/ signed by parent

　　　　　 _____ Classroom staff trained on Int. Swallow/ Emergency Plan

　　　　　 _____ Safe feeding/emergency plan initiated

　　　　　 _____ CAAB contacted (for behavioral feeding)

　　　　　 _____ Preconference held (behavior feeding)

DATE	PROCEDURE
_____	IEP meeting held (check attendance)

Persons attending:

☐ Teacher ☐ IEP facilitator ☐ Administrator

☐ SLP ☐ Nurse ☐ PT

☐ OT ☐ Parents ☐ Other _____

Issues Addressed at IEP: (check issues addressed)

☐ Emergency plan ☐ Release of information

☐ Medical history ☐ Temporary feeding plan

☐ Referral to physician ☐ Special diet

_____ Swallow and Feeding Plan and Emergency Plan reviewed and revised

_____ Training is conducted (check and date)

☐ Emergency Plan _____

☐ Swallowing and Feeding Plan _____

_____ Medical information/referral from physician is requested (check and date)

☐ MBSS _____ ☐ FEES _____

_____ Study conducted (attended by case manager)

        _____ IEP reconvened to update information

        _____ School personnel and parents trained in revised feeding plan

        _____ Revised feeding/treatment plan initiated

_____ Prescription for School Meal Modification is sent to/received from physician

_____ Prescription for School Meal Modification is faxed to food service supervisor

_____ School cafeteria manager and case manager review meal calendar and set up meal plan for student.

_____ Diet change started at school

_____ Therapy and swallowing treatment plan developed/ classroom staff and parents trained

Note. Printed with permission from the St. Tammany Parish Schools Special Education Department (2015).

APPENDIX J
Communication With Medical Providers Tool

Student's Name: _____

Date: _____

School Dysphagia Team Member's Name & Contact
Information:

_____

_____

School Dysphagia Team's Concerns Regarding Patient's
Feeding & Swallowing Skills:

_____

_____

_____

_____

_____

School Dysphagia Team has noticed the following
compensations/changes to assist the student during feeding:

_____

_____

_____

_____

_____

Please provide your professional opinion and comment on the following aspects of physiology and/or treatment options in the official report:

_____

_____

_____

_____

_____

Please contact me at the number below if you have questions on the day of the exam. If parent signs a release of information, please send the official report from today's assessment to the address listed below. Thank you,

_____

_____

Name: _____

Phone Number: _____

Address to Send Report: _____

APPENDIX K

School-Based Swallowing and Feeding Team Daily Feeding Log

Date: _____

Student: _____

School: _____

Time	Meal	Foods Offered	Foods Consumed	Liquids Offered	Liquids Consumed
___ to ___	Breakfast				
___ to ___	Snack				
___ to ___	Lunch				
___ to ___	Snack				

Note. Printed with permission from the St. Tammany Parish Schools Special Education Department (2015).

Index

Note: Page numbers in **bold** reference non-text material.

A

Abdominal cavity, 110
Academic performance, nutrition effects on, 49
ADA. *See* Americans with Disabilities Act
Adenoids, 113–114
Administrator, swallowing and feeding team, 27–31
Alveolar ducts, 109
Alveolar pressure, 110
Alveoli, 109
American Nurses Association Code of Ethics, 252–253
American Occupational Therapy Association Code of Ethics, 252–253
American Speech-Language-Hearing Association
Code of Ethics of, 55–56, 58
diet modifications, 215
dysphagia as defined by, 2
Americans with Disabilities Act, 52–53
Ankyloglossia, 113
Applied behavioral analysis, 196–197
Arytenoids, **116**
Aspiration
definition of, 108
dysphagia as cause of, 124, 130
pulmonary, 124
signs and symptoms of, 120, 124
Aspiration lung disease, 124

B

Barium swallow studies. *See* Modified barium swallow studies
BCBA. *See* Board certified behavior analyst
Behavioral feeding disorders
applied behavioral analysis approach to, 196–197
behaviors associated with, 175
characteristics of, 172–173
classroom teacher reports about, 175–176
definition of, 174
description of, 51, 62
four-tier hierarchy classification model for disordered feeders, **189**, 195–198
picky eaters, **189**, 190–192
proactive/prevention, 188–190, **189**
problem feeders, **189**, 192–195
schematic diagram of, **189**
summary of, 198

301

Food *(continued)*
  presentation of, 143
  types to avoid, 163–164, 168
Food diary, 161
Food log, 224, 299–300
Food safety, 168
Food service operations, in
  schools, 52
Free and appropriate public
  education, 9, 34, 41, 44, 173
Functional behavioral analysis, 62
Functional residual capacity, 110

G

Garrett case. *See Cedar Rapids*
  Community School v.
  Garrett F.
Gas exchange, 109
Gastroesophageal reflux, 182
Gastroesophageal reflux disease,
  117, 124
GERD. *See* Gastroesophageal
  reflux disease
Guardian(s). *See also* Family
  at-home swallowing and
    feeding skills established
    by, 242, 244
  of behavioral feeding disorder
    children, 174–175
  communication with, 90,
    238–239
  interview with
    description of, 90–91
    form used in, 90, 178, 221,
      271–276
  meals provided by, 214–215
  school district help and
    support for, 237–244
  swallowing and feeding team
    and
    concerns and issues, 31
    education, 237
    interview, **88**, 90–91

roles, 77–78, **86**, 91
validating the guardian's
  perspectives, 239–240
validating the perspective of,
  239–240

H

Health plan, individualized. *See*
  Individualized health plan
Heimlich maneuver
  description of, 3
  in individualized health plan, 93
  training in, 22
Hospitalization, 230
Hot dogs, 165
Hydration, 10, 216–226

I

IDEA. *See* Individuals with
  Disabilities Education
  Improvement Act of 2004
IEP. *See* Individualized education
  program
Individualized education plan,
  89, 95–96
Individualized education program
  adherence to, 62
  documentation regarding
    provision of, 63
  health care plan with, 50
  present level of academic
    achievement and
    functional performance,
    50
  school health services in, 44–45
Individualized health plan
  description of, 50, 61–62, 79
  review, revision, or retraining
    of, after individualized
    education plan
    conference, **89**, 99
  school nurse's preparation of, 93

Liquids
  school staff training in
    alterations of, 146
  thickening of, 151
Lower esophageal sphincter, 119
Lower respiratory tract, 108–109
Lungs
  anatomy of, 108–109
  gas exchange in, 109

M

Main stem bronchi, 109
Malnutrition, 217
Malocclusion, 113
Massage, oral, 152
Mastication, 118
MBSS. *See* Modified barium
    swallow studies
Meal(s). *See also* Diet; Food;
    Nutrition
  modifications to
    description of, **89**, 99–101
    form for, 100, 289–291
  parent/guardian provided,
    214–215
  school-provided. *See* School
    meals
  structuring of times for, 164
  student positioning during,
    142–143
Mechanical muscle response
    exercises, 152
Medicaid, 53–54, 59, 130
Medical records, 61
Medical services
  case law regarding, 45–46
  definition of, 44
  school health services versus,
    44–46
Medical settings, 4–6, **7**
Medical-based team
  description of, 36
  members of, 72–73

school-based team and,
    interactions between, 97,
    231
Medically fragile students. *See*
    Progressive disorders or
    medically fragile students
Modified barium swallow studies
  description of, 22, 30, 126
  goals of, 126
  referral for, 97–98
Mouth, 112–113

N

NASN. *See* National Association
    of School Nurses
Nasogastric tube feeding,
    157–158, 221
Nasopharynx, 114
National Association of School
    Nurses, 50
National School Lunch Act, 204
National School Lunch Program,
    51–52, 203–205, 225
No Child Left Behind Act, 41
Nurses. *See* School nurses
Nutrition. *See also* Diet;
    Food; School meals;
    Undernutrition
  academic performance affected
    by, 49
  body weight measurements to
    assess, 224
  cultural considerations,
    224–225
  daily feeding log for
    monitoring of, 224,
    299–300
  description of, 51–52
  importance of, 10
  information sources on, 190
  monitoring of, 224
  National School Lunch Program,
    51–52, 203–205, 225